Bedpans and Backrubs:

The Trials and Joys of a Student Nurse (1950-1953)

By: Marilyn Joyce Minter Wolgemuth

Copyright © 2017 by Marilyn Joyce Minter Wolgemuth

All rights reserved, including the right to reproduce the book or portions thereof in any form or by any means, electronic or mechanical, including photocopying, recording, or by any information storage and retrieval system, without permission in writing from the publisher. All inquiries should be addressed to Crave Press.

Printed in the United States of America

FIRST EDITION

ISBN: 978-0-9852599-9-0

Published by:
Crave Press
www.cravepress.com

What people are saying about this book:

"When I first heard the title of this book, Bedpans and Backrubs, I knew I was in for an honest, entertaining read about Marilyn's time in nursing school; and I wasn't disappointed. I was amazed to see how much has changed in terms of nursing education but also how much has changed for women. But more so than that historical overview, I enjoyed the personal side of the story. I saw Marilyn and her friends transform from students to graduate nurses, and I got to experience their honest trials, tribulations, and heartaches along the way. Despite the intense curriculum and expectations placed on nursing students and despite the ups and downs of school and hospital work, Marilyn's joy is evident throughout the entire book – she dreamed of being a nurse since she was 11 years old and the joy of living that dream never left her during her 65 years in nursing and beyond. This book is a must-read for anyone who wants to laugh, cry, and be inspired to find their calling and joy in life." Christina J. Steffy, Manager, Library Support Services, Education Innovation at Pennsylvania College of Health Sciences

This autobiographical account reads at times like a novel with some suspense: will she finish the training? Will she marry her boyfriend? Thanks to Marilyn's copious journals we learn what nursing education and hospitals, especially psychiatric hospitals, were really like sixty years ago. Lola Schmidt, proofreader.

Dedication

To my student nurse colleagues who agonized and also rejoiced with me through these three years of sweat and tears. I lovingly dedicate this account of our journey to become registered nurses.

Acknowledgments

I want to thank the following who have been helpful in bringing this book into being: Christina J. Steffy, manager of library support services, Pennsylvania College of Health Sciences, who enthusiastically evaluated the content for accuracy; Harold J. Eager who provided vital information about how Lancaster General Hospital and school of nursing evolved to what it is today in the commemorative book "One Hundred Years of Caring – Lancaster General Hospital"; John Enderle, director of LGH Alumni relations, Pennsylvania College of Health Sciences; Laurie Oswald Robinson, my diligent writing coach who edited the manuscript and who cheered me on through thick and thin; members of my writing group, Kathy Wiens and Kathy Goering, who graciously critiqued my initial efforts and provided helpful suggestions; Patrice Flaming APRN, my nurse friend who clarified how today's nurses are educated; Lola Schmidt, my exacting proofreader; and the helpful editors at Crave Press. Last but not least, the faithful faculty and my dear nursing student colleagues, you know who you are, who commiserated with me when the going was rough and rejoiced with me when happier times came along.

Bedpans and Backrubs:
The Trials and Joys of a Student Nurse (1950-1953)

By: Marilyn Joyce Minter Wolgemuth

Table of Contents

Prologue
Introduction

Part One: Six Months on Probation
Chapter 1 – Getting Acquainted
Chapter 2 – Classes and Heavy Studies Begin
Chapter 3 – Learning about Our Bodies
Chapter 4 – Working with Patients
Chapter 5 – Leisure Activities
Chapter 6 – Giving Medications
Chapter 7 – Dealing with Death and Dying
Chapter 8 – Women's Surgical Ward

Part Two: Six Months as a Junior Student
Chapter 9 – Our Capping Ceremony
Chapter 10 – Operating Room Experience
Chapter 11 – Men's Medical Ward / Evening Duty
Chapter 12 – Personal Sickness, Moving and Vacation
Chapter 13 – The Diet Kitchen

Part Three: Becoming Intermediate Nurses
Chapter 14 – Taking Another Big Step: The First Black Band for our Caps
Chapter 15 – Night Duty on Men's Surgical Ward
Chapter 16 – Women's Medical Ward
Chapter 17 – Beginning Maternity, Nursery, Labor and Delivery Rotation
Chapter 18 – Pediatric Ward and Polio Unit
Chapter 19 – Back to work at LGH

Part Four: One Year as Senior Students

Chapter 20 – Second Black Velvet Band for Our Caps
Chapter 21 – Psychiatric Rotation
Chapter 22 – Return to LGH
Chapter 23 – Emergency Room Rotation
Chapter 24 – The Final Countdown to Graduation
Chapter 25 – Dental Surgery and Goodbye to the Books
Chapter 26 – Graduation and Vacation
Chapter 27 – Apartment Hunting
Chapter 28 – Employed in Labor and Delivery; State Boards
Chapter 29 – Start New Job; Receiving License

Poem
Ode to an Embossed Piece of Paper:
Letting Go of My Nursing License

Epilogue

Appendix 1 – Nursing Education Today
Appendix 2 – Men Join the Nursing Profession
Appendix 3 – Current Information about Lancaster General Hospital and the Pennsylvania College of Health Sciences

Prologue

This book just begged to be written! As I reviewed all the journals that I wrote, I realized that they described in colorful detail my struggle with the rigors of a hospital-based, three-year diploma program. The following vignettes are based on the voluminous journals and letters I wrote while I was a student nurse. They graphically portray the way professional nurses were educated in 1950-1953. Much about nursing education has changed since then, as have almost all facets of the medical profession.

The excerpts from my actual journals and letters appear in italics. Most names of people and places have been changed to protect individuals' privacy. My young-adult writing style may seem rather naïve to some readers but my hope is that readers will get the flavor of what was involved in becoming a professional nurse in that era.

This type of nursing program was often referred to as "nurses' training." Since we train animals but we educate people I prefer to use the term nursing school instead. The program described in this narrative involved three full years of intensive classes, exams and extensive hands-on experiences in each of the different clinical specialties.

As students we were scheduled to rotate to all departments of the big city hospital. We spent several weeks or months at a time in each department learning to care for a variety of patients in different settings: medical, surgical, maternity, newborn and premature infant nursery, labor and delivery, surgery/operating rooms, pediatrics, orthopedics, EENT (eye, ear, nose and throat), polio, emergency room, diet kitchen, outpatient clinics, and psychiatry.

Probationers, Junior, Intermediate, and Senior nursing students were all expected to accept jumbled and erratic work schedules plus heavy study and classes. Classes were often scheduled on our one day off a week. We playfully called this rigorous unpaid work-study program "slave labor," a term we thought perfectly described all that was required of us.

When the probationary period was over, we worked 48 long, tiring hours a week on the wards to give the best possible patient care. All this was in addition to heavy classes and study. In our senior year we were granted a bit of relief when the government mandated a 44 hour work week.

Along with clinical bedside care, our instructors taught us a strict professional protocol of deference to doctors. If a nurse was sitting down when a doctor walked into the room, she was expected to rise and stand up as long as he was in the room. This practice may be discontinued in most of today's medical milieu where medical personnel collaborate more as academic equals.

I give my nursing instructors and ward supervisors a lot of credit for their personal interest in and patience with each of us. Their guidance and encouragement helped us to endure the tears and trials, hard work, and brain-drain that ultimately rewarded us with a well-deserved, excellent education.

Marilyn Minter Wolgemuth, Class of 1953
February 2016

Introduction

The first pinkish streaks of dawn greeted me. A cloudless, cerulean blue sky, a hint of autumn in the air, and a brisk early morning breeze signaled that fall weather was just around the corner. A vagrant breezes toyed lazily with the dry leaves that collected and swirled on the street in front of the house where I was staying. I awoke at 6 a.m. shivering with a mixture of excitement, fear, and uncertainty.

My friend dropped me off mid-morning and wished me well in my new endeavor. At last, my long-awaited nursing career was about to begin. As a starry-eyed 19-year-old country girl fresh from the Kansas prairies, I had anticipated this day for many moons.

My excitement was at a feverish pitch and my heart beat crazily as I gazed up at the tall, forbidding, gray concrete walls of this huge five-story building – Lancaster General Hospital School of Nursing (LGH).

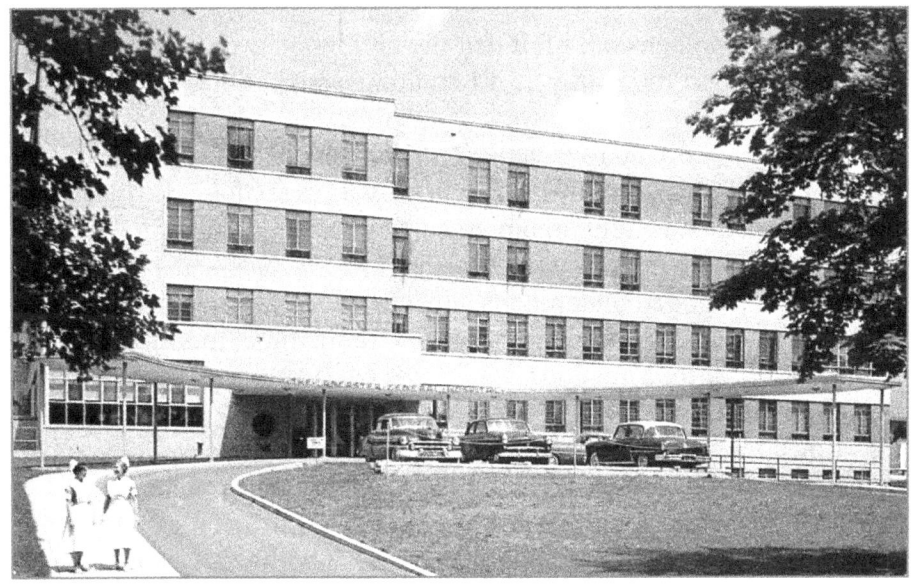

Lancaster General Hospital School of Nursing, 1952

This would be my sanctuary for the next three years, from September 1950 through September 1953. I knew I was ready to tackle the rigorous journey through these hushed halls of learning. I just didn't know how rigorous the journey would be.

Fifty five young women on the cusp of adulthood were poised to embark on this tumultuous, uncharted journey to become nurses. All of us trembled with nervous apprehension.

As I joined the registration line, I thought, "what am I getting myself into?" Next to me in line was a student wearing a name tag, "Heidi," She seemed just as nervous as I was. She restlessly twirled her dark brown hair with her one hand and bit her fingernails to the quick on the other hand. "Maybe we could comfort each other", I thought.

"I'm beginning to wonder if this is what I signed up for!" I said aloud to Heidi.

Heidi replied in a quivery voice, "Me, too! I'm scared to death!"

"Well, it's a little too late to back out now," I said.

"I know. Let's hope we can tough it through," she replied.

Despite my apprehension, I felt that my childhood dream of becoming a nurse could become reality….if I could just stick it out.

The seeds of my dream to be a nurse were first planted in my heart when I was 11 years old. In 1942, when I was in sixth grade, I had an emergency appendectomy in our small-town hospital, the same hospital where my birth mother had died in 1934. She had a painful death from a ruptured gangrenous appendix due to misdiagnosis by the country doctor. I was only three years old at the time, totally unaware of the gravity of the situation.

This time around my father took extreme precautions to avoid a repeat of that grievous experience. He didn't want that same outcome to happen to his beloved daughter. Ignoring the extravagant expense, he hired Miss Winter to be my 24-hour private duty nurse. He wanted me to have the best care possible. Happily, I had an uncomplicated recovery.

I absolutely loved the personal, professional care Miss Winter gave me. By the time I left the hospital, I knew what I wanted to do when I grew up – care for others in the same gentle way. Strong, unmistakable compassion began to stir within me. My new interest prompted me to read everything I could about nursing which included all of the "Cherry Ames" nurse books that I checked out of our small town public library – flight nurse, emergency nurse, private duty nurse, cruise nurse, etc. My insatiable appetite for each book further fueled my desire to go into the nursing profession.

When my girlfriends came to play at my home on Sunday afternoons, we often played "doctor" with the doctor kit I received for my 12th birthday. At age 15, I begged my Aunt Mary to loan me the correspondence course she had taken years before. I devoured that heavy 600 page volume, A Home Nursing Textbook. All through high school I took science courses to further prepare myself.

After graduation from high school, I attended Messiah College near Harrisburg, Pennsylvania, for two years, our church's denominational junior college. I enrolled in the pre-nursing courses in order to be better qualified for entrance into nursing school. By the time I graduated from Messiah in 1950 with an A.A. degree, all my Kansas peers had also left home to pursue their careers so there was nothing to entice me to return to Kansas.

I decided to choose a nursing school in Pennsylvania so I could stay in touch with the many good friends I made at Messiah. A budding romance with a native Pennsylvanian, a handsome guy named Carl, began several months before graduation; that was another compelling reason for staying in PA. Would our relationship survive the ups and downs of a three year courtship with me in nursing school and him in college? It was a risk we would take. Only time would tell.

Part One

Six Months on Probation

Chapter 1
Getting Acquainted

September 10, 1950: *This was truly a red-letter day - the biggest, scariest, most thrilling step of my life lay ahead of me as I joined the students who were in line for registration. I didn't know a soul. But that would soon change.*

With registration over, Miss Becket, a plump, soft-spoken lady with a blonde pageboy hair style, directed us to a classroom where we waited for further instructions. In a smooth, encouraging tone of voice, she explained that our class had now launched on a period of probation. She informed us that for the next six months we would be called "probies". During the probation period the faculty would assess each student's ability to handle the work schedule and class material. In March, if all went well, we would receive our student caps and become junior students.

"We know each of you will do your best," she added comfortingly at the end of her speech.

A little voice inside me said, "Okay, here we go! Sock it to me. I am ready to take it on!"

Learning Lesson #1

September 11, 1950: *After a hearty lunch in the cafeteria, we returned to the classroom. Miss B divided us into five groups of eleven students. Each instructor took her group on a guided tour through the entire hospital. No one talked very much as we shuffled along behind our leaders. It would be safe to say that we were all experiencing similar emotions of awe, anxiety, and apprehension.*

As my group traipsed through Men's Surgical Ward, an elderly man dropped his lighted cigarette onto the paper in the metal wastebasket by his bed. The paper quickly caught on fire and flared close to the bed sheet dangling over the basket. Miss Burt, the instructor, quickly grabbed the wastebasket away from the bed and frantically yelled to the nurse who was charting in the nurses station close by, "Hey, Miss Kenna, quick! Bring water to douse this fire! Hurry!"

Miss Kenna came running with a pail of water and extinguished the fire before it could spread further. She scolded the man in a voice loud enough to wake up napping patients. "Mr. Bates, you know better than to throw a lighted cigarette in the wastebasket. You could have burned down the whole hospital!"

His face flushed and he apologized profusely, "Oh, I'm so sorry, Miss. All these lovely young ladies distracted me so much that I did it without thinking."

The nurse detected a sly grin on his wrinkled face. She struggled to keep a straight face herself as she said ruefully, "Next time, don't let a pretty girl distract you when you have a lighted cigarette in your hand."

I mused more to myself than anyone else, "Maybe it won't be so hard after all."

This was our lesson #1 – how do deal with an arsonist!

A few of the girls thought they could try the program on for size to see if they were cut out to be nurses. Several others said they viewed nursing as a glamorous profession that could pull in a comfortable salary. The majority of us entered into the program wholly dedicated to serve people in need of compassionate care. This area of Pennsylvania was heavily populated with church-affiliated people so a large percentage of the entire student body was connected with local churches.

Throughout the three years we were inundated with:

- grueling heavy-duty, study-intensive classes,
- six to eight weeks of clinical rotations on each patient ward,
- sixteen weeks in maternity, labor and delivery,
- twelve weeks in a psychiatric rotation,
- weird work and class schedules,

- precious days off cancelled or changed,
- grumpy and pleasant patients,
- chronic weariness,
- sleep deprivation,
- mood swings,
- dorm pranks,
- tough exams,
- frustrations,
- romantic joys and woes,
- new friends and roommates,
- competition for study space in cramped dorm rooms,
- low points of threatening to quit the program,
- high points of accomplishments!

If we had known everything that loomed ahead at the beginning, I daresay many of us would have chickened out, called it quits, picked up our books and headed home in defeat. As it turned out, all but four of us persevered to the very end.

Enduring the heat of the first months

Our class was one of the largest in the 57-year history of the school of nursing. Housing resources were stretched to the max in four different nurses' residences near the hospital. I was assigned to Fraim House, a decaying, turn-of-the-century, dark-grayish house with peeling paint. There was no central air, only windows that opened to let in the humid air in spring and summer. An ancient, coal-fed furnace that belched coal dust and spat flames would barely heat the whole house in the winter.

Ten of my classmates were assigned rooms on the two lower levels. Jean, Melanie, and I were assigned to the third floor. The three of us climbed up the rickety stairs to a drab attic room directly under the non-insulated roof.

"I'm depressed already!" I murmured to myself, hoping no one would hear me complain this early in the game. "How are we supposed to study in this dump?"

Another girl overheard me and quipped, "At least we have a roof over our heads until it leaks when it rains!"

Everyone sweltered and sweated from the suffocating humidity and high September temperatures. The three of us felt the heat most intensely as it radiated through the roof of our top floor room.

It was useless to gripe about our circumstances – complaining only depressed us more. I found at least one positive thing about living here. The most important destinations were close by. The cafeteria, classrooms, and hospital work assignments were conveniently located directly across the street.

That evening, we munched on sugar cookies and sipped ice-cold ginger ale as we sat in a circle on the living room floor for a get-acquainted session. It was fun to pick nicknames for each other, too. Usually it was some form of our first or last names. Since my last name was Minter they dubbed me "Minnie" right away (that stuck with me throughout the whole time).

Chapter 2
Classes and Heavy Studies Begin

The next day classes and a heavy study schedule began, starting with A&P (anatomy and physiology), nursing arts, chemistry, pharmacology, and microbiology. We were relentlessly inundated with textbooks.

We learned resourcefulness and how to get along with a minimum of simple supplies and equipment. Many of the complicated medical procedures, high-tech medical equipment, and dizzying array of pills for every pain that are available today were non-existent in 1950.

Plastic items were not yet in vogue so there were no disposable or pre-sterilized materials. Glass syringes, hypodermic needles, IV tubing, rubber catheters, and surgical instruments were either boiled or autoclaved for 30 minutes to one hour. Glass thermometers were sterilized by soaking them in alcohol in rectangular metal trays. Before putting a glass thermometer under a patient's tongue for three minutes, we gingerly and gently wiped the alcohol off with a cotton ball.

In nursing arts class, we learned many new procedures. We practiced giving injections first by plunging a needle into an orange and later on each other, giving a relaxing backrub to soothe a patient, and making perfect "hospital corners" on a patient's bed sheets that had to pass meticulous inspection by fussy instructors.

We also learned how to comfortably place and remove a bed pan under a patient, deep-clean and sterilize the bedpans, give an enema, catheterize a patient, and feed a helpless patient. We practiced taking blood pressures, pulses, and respirations on each other. We learned the importance of washing our hands between each patient.

Since there were no disposable sterile supplies available as there are today, we:

made our own Q-tips by wrapping part of a cotton ball on long toothpicks then sterilized packets of them in an ancient autoclave that shuddered and shook during the whole process;

sterilized the glass syringes, needles, and surgical instruments in a water boiler or autoclave for 30 minutes or more;

used the hypodermic needles over and over, checking each one carefully after several uses to see if it had developed a "hook" on the end due to repeated use. To do this, we dragged the needle over a cotton ball to see if it snagged a wisp of cotton. If it did, our job was to hone the hook on a small whetstone until the needle was perfectly smooth and sharp again when tested with a cotton ball. It must be able to penetrate a patient's skin with the least amount of trauma, otherwise it would feel like we were driving a dull knife into the patient thus increasing the pain; and wrapped bandages made from worn sheets.

September 14, 1950: *Our first assignment in anatomy and physiology lab was to prick our fingers and examine our blood under the microscope. This grossed out several of the girls. Becky fainted at the sight of her own blood but we soon revived her with smelling salts. [Smelling salts contain ammonium carbonate and perfume; they give off a strong odor designed to hit the olfactory nerves with a bang and revive an unconscious person when placed under the nose.]*

Heidi's face turned ashen as she whined, "Ugh, I can't stand the sight of blood either! I'm going to puke!"

I rushed with her to the bathroom where she vomited. She soon managed to pull herself together and go on with the class, although she was quite emotionally shaken. She apologized for being so squeamish. I gently reassured her that she would soon get used to seeing blood. It is just part of being a nurse. I grew up on a farm where we butchered beef and chickens, so I was accustomed to seeing lots of blood!

September 20, 1950: *Carl called me on the pay phone for the first time this evening. It sent a thrill through my body because it had been two weeks since we had seen each other. He was in a cheery mood and it was so good to hear his voice. I really miss the college milieu and sometimes feel homesick for all my friends there.*

He asked what the weather was like here. I fought a brief wave of irritation that his first concern was the weather instead of how things were going for me. When I described our hot third floor room, he wondered if I could request another place to live. I told him rooms were so scarce we'll just have to put up with it.

Before he hung up he told me, "Marilyn, don't let the hospital take away your sweetness! I miss you."

"OK, I promise not to complain so much! I miss you, too! Bye, for now."

I hung up the phone and ran for the box of Kleenex. My tears flowed freely as a wave of nostalgia and homesickness swept over me.

Some of my fellow nurses were so "boy crazy" they couldn't stand being cooped up and required to be in every night with a 10 p.m. curfew. What really made them hopping mad were two more hard and fast rules:

1) Anyone who flunks a test must forfeit the one overnight privilege a month,

2) A student could neither enter nor remain in the program if she were married or pregnant.

Most nursing schools prior to 1970 had that second rule. That was difficult for the girls with steady boyfriends. One of them dropped out because she couldn't wait to get married.

The glitz and glamor rubs off

We were a determined bunch of young women. It wasn't long, though, before the glitz and glamor wore very thin and at times our spirits sagged dangerously low. The heavy studies gradually sapped our physical and emotional energy. The first six months period of probation would tell how many of the 55 "eager beavers" would hang in there through it all. Later we had to cope with the exhausting hours of work on the hospital wards.

Eating and studying, studying and eating

It seemed like all we did was eat and study, study and eat, then study some more. If we were lucky, we might get a few hours of sleep. Most evenings I holed up in my room and pounded anatomy and physiology into my brain for our first tough test at the end of September. Luckily, I studied the right things and got passing grades on the tests. The next three weeks passed by so quickly.

September 25, 1950: I aired some of my feelings in a long letter to Carl:

Life is really getting interesting here. It's so much fun to learn the intricacies of the human body. Classes go clear through the day. I'm enjoying every minute of it, so far. I made 91 in pharmacology and that is a very exacting course. I made 88 on the anatomy and physiology test last week. Not the best grade, but hopefully it will get better.

I pulled the most stupid "boner" today in microbiology class when Mrs. Wentz took me off guard. She asked me "Miss Minter, what is the opposite of 'biogenesis'?" I innocently answered, "spontaneous combustion." You should have heard the class roar with laughter! Even Mrs. Wentz herself nearly split laughing. I should have said "spontaneous generation"! I was thinking the word but combustion came out instead.

Tonight at the supper table the girls teased me mercilessly by calling me "Little Miss Spontaneous Combustion." I don't think I'll ever live that one down! That was the corniest mistake I've made in a long time. It won't be the last, either.

Yesterday was such a drizzly day. Even though the skies were weeping and the sun had tucked itself away for the day, I could play the piano in the parlor and sing "I have sunshine in my heart today." Carl, I just feel like bubbling some happiness over your way right now! Guess I'd better get back to studying for tomorrow's test. I'll be like an artist and "draw this letter to a close." Bye, Marilyn.

September 30, 1950: *Today Miss Becket showed us the ghastly, sickly blue, saggy, baggy smocks we were expected to wear when we start working with patients on the wards. Those horrid things billow out like maternity smocks that make us look pregnant. We figure that Miss Keeger ordered such ridiculous things for us to wear so the patients will laugh when they see us and get well quicker! Laughter is supposed to be the best medicine, as the saying goes. This I must see.*

On the positive side, though, Miss B told us the hospital will launder our uniforms so that's one less thing we have to worry about. It is important to find something for which, to be thankful if we are to stay sane and optimistic in this place.

In six weeks we will turn in those hated smocks and receive the regular blue-and-white striped student uniforms with white starched collars and bib-less aprons. That's right no bibs yet! Without bibs on our aprons, we will easily be identified as probies. The bibs will be issued in March when we receive our student nurses' caps at the capping ceremony and become juniors. This was the first I'd ever heard of having to work for the privilege of wearing a bib!

Finding friends and homes away from home

Since my parents lived several hundred miles away, I couldn't visit them on a regular basis. Several local families invited me to hang out with them on my days off, especially the Grove and the Harden families. I appreciated their hospitality and always felt so welcome. They invited me to help with cooking, baking, gardening, and processing garden produce. And we played games just like I would do with my own family if they lived closer. My friends often sent enough food back with me to share with my housemates. Party time!

My three closest friends in the student program were Gracie, Molly and Naomi. Each of them had such a different personality. We had many good times together.

Gracie was a fun-loving, outgoing and spiritually mature senior nursing student, an excellent example of a dedicated nurse. She and I developed a very close emotional bond and often did extracurricular activities together. I went to her when I was discouraged and ready to tear my hair out over the tough tests, classes or some minor kerfuffle with staff, patients or colleagues. Her goal was to be a missionary nurse in Africa. She later spent several years at a mission hospital teaching student nurses in Zambia, Africa.

Molly had an exuberant, vivacious personality, an infectious laugh and a non-stop zest for life! She started in the nursing program the year after I did, and we became close like soul-sisters. We often came up with the most adventurous, daring and sometimes risky things to do on our days and weekends off duty. Her family lived at the outskirts of Elizabethtown, 30 minutes away, and their home became my home away from home. They "adopted" me and I was so grateful to have a substitute family since my own family lived far away. Dependable bus service was available to Elizabethtown so I often spent my days off with Molly's family.

Naomi was three years older than me, very shy, quiet, and studious with a warm generous smile. We had been in the same college class. She and I shared a room our last two years. We got along well together even though we were so different. Sometimes, she invited me to go with her to her home 10 miles away when we had the same days off duty.

Moving, and moving again!

At the beginning of November, the director of nursing notified my roommates and me that we were to move to another nurses' residence; our attic room on the third floor would be too cold in winter. That was good news, but I wondered, why hadn't all the smart people around here figured that out before we moved in? I think all 55 of us must have descended on them so fast before they were completely ready for us. In a strange way, though, I hated to leave this rickety place. In these two months I had come to love this old Fraim House with all its drafty crevices, creaks and groans.

Jean and Melanie moved across the street to Forney House and assured me they would help me move when it was my turn. A few days later, they were as good as their word. I moved my meager belongings to another rather ancient structure, the Duke Street residence a block away. It was an old but sturdy brick house, and it was better insulated.

Surprise! A week after I was cozily settled there the housemother announced that someone had messed up the moving schedule and I was supposed to move to Forney House instead! So, I packed up my stuff and moved…again.

What was the bright side of all this upheaval? Forney House is more modern so I didn't complain. Variety is the spice of life, they say, so I must learn to be flexible and realize everything doesn't always go my way. Wow, what a philosopher I was getting to be!

October 15, 1950: *My new roomie Ruthie and I have very different personality types, so it will be a stretch for both of us to live together in such close proximity. Ruthie is gracious, studious, reserved, and shy. I am also studious, but tend to be impulsive, moody, outgoing, and opinionated.*

She grew up in a religious community that wasn't as legalistic as the very conservative church community where I had grown up. I am quite naïve about how to live in close quarters with someone who has a different religious experience. It won't take long though until we get to know each other and live happily together.

Writing helps me relax and sort out my feelings about each day's activities. Every night, before I go off to sleep in la-la land, I pray and read my Bible and then pull out my trusty journal from its hiding place under the mattress. There is so little privacy in this place that I don't know who might snoop around trying to find it.

One day the hospital cafeteria served carrot salad with delicious chopped dates. Mimi, a rather stout girl, solemnly announced, "I'm going to eat only carrot salad since that isn't fattening."

I quickly informed her, "The dates in the salad are fattening!"

Witty friend Jane caught me on that one and laughingly teased me, "Is that why you gain weight after you have a date with Carl, Minnie?" I must have blushed profusely and giggled girlishly along with the others. They obviously enjoyed teasing me with that spice of life.

Chapter 3
Learning about Our Bodies

November 1, 1950: *Never have I realized until today how utterly miraculous our bodies are! When we study the detailed and complex composition of all our systems, I have no doubt about the omnipotence of the Creator! I just have to marvel at how our circulatory, digestive, respiratory and all the rest of our body systems are so complete and intricate. I wouldn't give up this wonderful experience for anything! Learning all about our bodies boosts my faith and just simply fascinates me.*

November 15, 1950: *I just found out that 33 of our class flunked the anatomy and physiology test over the skeletal system last week, and all of them had to forfeit their overnight privileges this week. I pity them just a wee bit but maybe they could help themselves if they would only study a little bit harder and not party so much!*

Here's the list of tough tests coming up the next few days: the midterm in psychology, a unit test in nursing arts, the big chemistry test on Thursday. Friday is another big one in A & P over the muscle system. Wow! That is tough sledding. All I've done the last two weeks is study for tests. But truthfully I'm fascinated with every one of my courses.

Once in a while we compare grades. If I get a better grade someone might needle me by saying, "You must be smarter because you went to college." I don't like when they say that because I'm not any smarter than the rest. Maybe I just choose to study harder, huh?

Discovering the anatomy of a big city hospital

What does a patient ward in a big city hospital look like? At LGH the wards consisted of long, unadorned rooms with tall, narrow windows along one side. Twelve single hospital beds six beds on each side of the room were about two feet apart. A couple of the wards had an additional sun room with two or four beds. Four or more private rooms were located on the other side of the nurses' station.

A bedside stand held each patient's personal hygiene items, a bath basin and, of course, the urinal or bedpan he or she used.

Adjacent to the wards were the small nurses' stations where we prepared medications and charted patients' progress. Across the hall from the nurses' station was a small kitchenette where we made simple snacks for the patients: toast, broth, crackers, tea, or coffee.

That many patients in close proximity to each other meant a nightly chorus of snoring, coughing, and wheezing which could be a major deterrent to a good night of sleep. Another disadvantage was that there was very little privacy for anyone. For a doctor's exam, dressing changes, bed baths, and toileting, the nurse would pull the heavy cloth curtain on a rod around the entire bed.

Separate wards on different floors of the hospital had specialized names and uses. Students were assigned to work eight-hour shifts - days, evenings and nights - in each of these departments for specified lengths of weeks or months during the three-year period.

Women's Medical, Men's Medical, Women's Surgical, Men's Surgical, EENT (Ear, Eye, Nose and Throat), Pediatrics, and Orthopedic wards as well as operating rooms and recovery rooms took up most of four floor. The Maternity section was in a separate wing of the hospital. It consisted of three floors of private and semi-private rooms for about 52 mothers. Labor and delivery rooms were on third floor of the maternity wing. In a nursery on each floor, special teams of nurses cared for newborns, including one for premature babies.

Emergency Rooms and Outpatient clinics were located in other areas of the hospital. The morgue/autopsy rooms were in the basement near the hospital exit. Thankfully we didn't have to work there, but it was necessary to go there to deliver the body of a patient who died.

In 1950, the average daily patient count in the hospital was 285 with a charge of $10.73 per day for ward beds, $12 per day for private rooms, and $9.50 per day for semi-private rooms. In 1951, rates went up to $12.06 per day. In 1952, a new addition added 156 new beds that brought the census up to a total of 456. At that time, the average patient stay was 12 days for medical-surgical patients and 7 days for maternity patients ("100 years of caring - Lancaster General Hospital," by Harold Eager 1994).

Learning to care for the dead and dying patient

I wrote another long letter to Carl:

Yesterday in the lecture for nursing arts class, Mrs. Long demonstrated the care of the critically ill, the dying, and the dead. She had us all shivering with chills of dread at the thought of performing the last duties on a dead person.

On Men's Medical Ward the nurses have what they call "Death Row", patients that are expected to clunk out at any minute. I doubt if it would take much for me to lie down and die alongside my first dying patient rather than face the stark horror of the death rattle and the glassy stare. Some morning I'll discover that I gave a patient his/her last back rub the night before. But it all goes with nursing. I must work with poise, dignity, and reserve and not let my feelings get in the way. Gotta sign off for now ... M

My journal continues: *One section of the class observed an autopsy yesterday. To hear them talk about it afterwards almost made my blood curdle. Out of curiosity, I'm eager to see one, though, when my turn comes around. Meanwhile, our group made slides of tubercle bacilli, mycobacteria, etc. How utterly boring!*

The next evening I wrote about my experience at the autopsy:
Today it was our turn. Ten of us stood around the autopsy table where a female's nude body was lying on the hard, cold steel slab. The medical examiner had opened up the abdomen and the intestines were all laid out where he could examine them. What a jolting sight that proved to be! I never dreamed anything could be so revolting, gruesome, and at the same time so fascinating.

The medical examiner doing the autopsy told us that the woman was a victim of chronic alcoholism, syphilis, gonorrhea, and possibly tuberculosis. The autopsy team did a complete dissection – brain and all – while we stood and watched, enthralled by all that we saw.

The smell of formaldehyde was almost overwhelming. It amazed me that not one student got sick to her stomach. It wouldn't have surprised me if someone had upchucked right there. It's just another instance where we must steel our emotions to the extent that nothing outwardly affects us. Sometimes I think I can feel myself emotionally hardening when I have to defend myself against the more unpleasant aspects of nursing.

Studying hard for tests

October 20, 1950: *Last week we got our papers back in psychology, and what a lot of groans when we discovered the highest grade was 83 and the lowest was 21. The professor talks so far beyond our level. We usually don't understand half of what he's talking about. I don't think any of us were shocked at the grades. When 90% of the class fails a test you know something must be screwy about the teacher. Thank goodness he grades on the curve.*

When I peeked at our psychology final this morning, I gasped in disbelief... four pages of sentence completion, essay, and multiple choices! It was inhumane and cruel, and it didn't even cover stuff that he had told us to study. [Later, I shouted for joy when I found out I passed it with an 82.]

Yesterday in anatomy, we dissected brains. What a gooey mess that was! For our inquisitive minds, though, it was extremely interesting to see what is inside the brain and learn a little bit more about that mass of gray matter in our cranial cavity.

I studied really hard for the microbiology test on Saturday morning. It is such a technical and complicated subject. Today the teacher posted our final grades, and she must have done some major juggling of grades because every one of us passed! We still don't understand how that could happen because several of the girls had flunked every test so far.

Chapter 4
Working with Patients

Working on the hospital wards

A month after we entered these hallowed halls, we worked our first two-hour floor duty on the wards. We didn't care for patients yet though. My buddies and I were assigned to do drudge work. We cleaned cupboards, wrapped sheet bandages, made cotton applicator swabs, and practiced getting a unit ready for the next admission.

October 7, 1950: *Here we are, mere probies, privileged to do all this dirty work. You'd think we were the janitors around here! These are not very exciting things to do, I agree. Our practical experience is still so limited, though. But I don't mind. Nearly every worthwhile occupation starts with lowly jobs.*

I was very eager to actually work with patients. We were scheduled to start by working only two hours at a time using skills we had practiced in class. These included giving bed-baths, backrubs, morning care, etc. It was good that tasks were introduced gradually and in short segments, otherwise we would have been overwhelmed. Our nursing supervisors were very patient with us.

I wrote again the next day: *Today was my first big chance to work directly with patients on Women's Medical Ward. The ward supervisor assigned two patients for me to give morning care. I helped them brush their teeth, change bed linens, and give bed-baths and backrubs. I was a bit nervous, but every minute of it was simply engrossing.*

My first patient was an elderly woman who had 22 teeth pulled yesterday and her mouth was in a pathetic condition. Teeth-brushing was not an option since she had no teeth. I tried to help her rinse out her mouth with diluted salt water. She couldn't get the hang of swishing it around in her mouth. She kept spitting it out along with blood. Yuck!

My second patient was tearful and needed some TLC – tender loving care. She had recently been diagnosed with cancer and was waiting for more testing. After her bath, I offered her one of my relaxing backrubs for which I am becoming rather famous. She, in turn, wanted me to have one of her sweet navel oranges fresh from sunny California. She thanked me profusely for helping her feel more relaxed.

October 20, 1950: *Today from 2-4 p.m. several of us gave afternoon care to patients on Women's Medical, one of the busiest wards: refill pitchers with fresh drinking water, offer nutritious liquids and, yes, give backrubs and special skin care. Most patients lie in bed for long periods of time, and their skin requires frequent stimulation to prevent painful and ugly pressure sores. Older peoples' tender skin is especially vulnerable to break down quickly if we don't give good skin care.*

I gave an enema to an obese female patient in preparation for tomorrow morning's scheduled abdominal surgery. She wasn't real happy about that procedure. She also complained about having to take only clear liquids by mouth after 6 p.m.

Bless her heart. I guess she wasn't too offended. She offered me chocolates from her ample supply in the bedside drawer. Ah, the generosity of patients and the rewards of being a nurse. Chocolates and oranges. It doesn't get much better than that!

Giving an enema was what I liked the least. And we gave so many of them! I had to use lots of tact and diplomacy to explain what I was about to do and persuade the patient to allow me to do it. Many times I had to soothe a person who considered it to be an invasive and humiliating experience.

Calming a restless patient with a relaxing backrub was what I found most satisfying. The patient usually gave a muffled sigh of satisfaction into the pillow and groaned with pleasure, "Ooh that feels so good!" With that I felt well paid. Soon I became known for my good backrubs.

[In today's hospital environment, patients don't spend as much time in bed. Instead they are encouraged to be ambulatory within 24 hours of surgical procedures. For that reason, backrubs have gone the way of the dinosaur for the most part.

I would like to see backrubs reinstated. In my experience of providing care for patients, I have found there is something about a gentle hands-on touch that is almost as powerful as a pain pill or muscle relaxant. Bedpans are not often needed either anymore because patients are encouraged to walk to the bathroom on their own as soon as possible after surgery or other procedure.]

It was always a thrill to practice a new skill on Mrs. Chase, the make-believe "patient"/mannequin that we practiced on every day. We learned a lot by practicing on her. She put up with our bumbling attempts to learn how to do various procedures; she never complained, though. Wouldn't it be nice if all patients would be so easy to work with?

One day Polly and I were working together in the utility room. She accidentally knocked over the blood transfusion tray and broke all the glass tubes in the process of cleaning cupboards. What a mess to clean up. I felt sorry for her. It could have easily happened to me. I could be real clumsy and all thumbs at times.

I commented that by this time next year the new batch of probies will be here and we can stand back and watch them slave away doing the dirty work around here like we do now. I tingled with glee when I thought of that prospect!

When Henrietta and I studied anatomy and physiology together one evening, we got into such a giggling mood. Needless to say, our study time was minimal. We ended up doing what she suggested – we put hot packs on our pimples.

Strutting our stuff

November 29, 1950: *Miss Becker issued the new blue and white striped uniforms with white starched collars and bib-less white wrap-around aprons that buttoned in the back. That's right, NO bibs! At last* *we could ditch those awful blue smocks. However, we could still easily be identified as "those probies with no bibs."*

Now we can wear our spiffy new uniforms and strut confidently down the hushed corridors just as the honorable juniors, intermediates, and seniors do. Starched skirts rustle, rubber soles and heels thump quietly on the tiled floor. We have definitely worked our way up the ladder a notch.

The first day wearing our new uniforms, both sides of my neck became painful when I turned my head. Upon examination, I saw that the stiff starched white collar rubbed my sternocleidomastoid muscles, relentlessly poked me under my jaw, and turned my skin a brilliant red!

My sternocleidomastoid – what does that big word mean? Hmm, that's a beautiful word from anatomy and physiology. It means the large muscles at the sides of the neck. I like big words like that. They run smoothly over my tongue like melted butter!

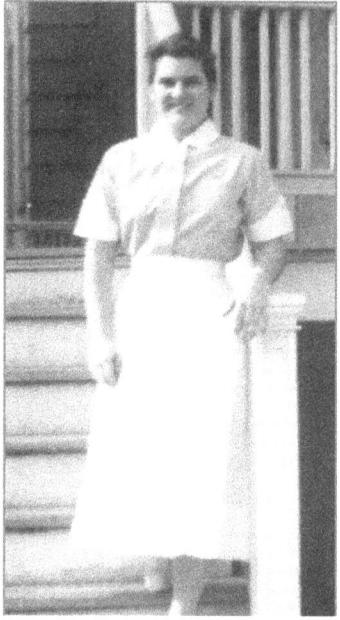

Marilyn in her student uniform

I have a hard time keeping my freshly polished shoes scrupulously white when I traipse through the slush as I cross the snowy street. Miss Keeger inspects all of us with her sharp eagle eyes each time before we go on duty. We line up in the classroom for inspection and she scolds us if our duty shoes aren't perfectly polished, if the seam on our white nylon stockings isn't straight or if anything else is amiss.

[After the six-month probation period was completed in March, and just before the capping ceremony, Mrs. K issued the bibs that we attached to the aprons. Each bib had the student's name embroidered in the upper left corner.]

December 4, 1950: *This afternoon I went downtown, walked into a store, approached a clerk, and told her what I wanted.*

The clerk looked at me rather strangely and then said, "You know, I could have spotted you a mile away."

That shocked and amazed me because I had never seen the clerk before. "Why do you say that?" I asked, hesitantly.

The clerk answered, "Well, you're a nurse aren't you?"

"Yes," I said, with a puzzled expression, wondering where this conversation was going.

"I thought so," said the clerk with a big toothy smile on her face. "I can usually tell a nurse by the way she walks."

I thought the woman must be a lunatic or something. I timidly ventured another question, "How do I walk?"

The clerk replied, "All you nurses have a characteristic walk – swift, steady and long steps. You look like you're going somewhere important."

I thought the whole conversation was so bizarre. Would I recognize a nurse when I see one walking down the street?

During the pleasantly warm weather, Dr. H. conducted one of our sociology classes outdoors on the lawn – a nice break from routine. Another day he took us to visit several social agencies – the Public Health Department, the Visiting Nurses Association, the Red Cross, and others. My group learned about Visiting Nurses Association and the Public Health Department. I was impressed as the instructor explained their methods and purposes. For a long time I had often thought being a visiting nurse would be a great opportunity. That day my desire to be a public health or visiting nurse became stronger than ever. That field seemed like it would fit me the best.

[My wish was granted when the Fresno County (CA) Health Dept. hired me in 1955 as one of the county public health nurses. I very much enjoyed teaching mother and baby classes, counseling patients who came to the weekly clinics, and making home visits in the many agricultural migrant camps on the county's west side.]

Starting the New Year with one less student

We all thought things were going along very smoothly until we got the news that one less student was in our ranks.

January 6, 1951: *I processed my sad feelings by journaling again: Last week, Patty was asked to quit the program. Poor girl, I felt so sorry for her. Mrs. K told her she'd have to leave due to her poor grades. How many more classmates will leave these sheltering walls before their wings are fully developed? I'm afraid others will want to quit, too. I've had similar temptations myself due to the heavy studies, the crazy working hours, and minimal social life. I just have to give myself a good pep talk and pray for God to help me through it.*

Then today all of us were dumbstruck again when Mrs. K informed us that Margie decided to quit the program and took her books home last night. She must have been very discouraged and didn't feel free to talk to anyone about her depressed feelings. Pangs of pain seared my heart until I almost cried. I felt so sad about losing her.

Waiting to become Junior students

January 11, 1951: *Earlier on this snowy evening, several of us nibbled snacks as we chatted in the parlor after classes were over for the day. Cindy and Marge rejoiced by pirouetting in the middle of the room, exclaiming that soon we would get our bibs and caps. In two more months we will become junior nursing students instead of mere probies. The days can't go fast enough for me. I wish the next two months would drop out of sight and it would be March 13.*

I live for the day the older students and graduates no longer look down their noses at us but instead treat us as equals. They are so quick to criticize us for the least little thing and saddle us with all the menial jobs. There is no guarantee they won't treat us that way even though we move up a notch. Who knows? I vow to be gentle and supportive of the new students who will be coming in September.

Starting to work four-hour shifts on Women's Medical

Up to this point we had worked only two-hour shifts at a time. Now we would double that and work four hours at a time.

February 15, 1951: *The patients on Women's Medical Ward welcomed four of us "probies" with open arms this morning. It was our first four-hour, 8 a.m.-12 noon, shift. Miss B, head nurse, had my patient assignments ready for me.*

Mrs. Achey was one of the patients on my list. What an appropriate name for a sick hospital patient, I thought. I groaned inwardly, though, when I saw her name on my work sheet. Other nurses have reported that she's so hard to please.

She has a huge abdominal hernia that is big enough to fill a medium sized washbowl. As she turns from one side to the other, she lifts the hernia up and over to her other side! It is dreadful to watch her do it. The doctors say they've never seen anything like it.

As I approached her bed, she let me know in no uncertain terms, "I don't want a bath now. Come back later!" I had been told that women are much fussier than men. Now I've come to believe it.

I decided to try engaging her in conversation. I asked about her family and then listened patiently as she talked about her troubles.

"My husband walked out on me last month, and a week ago my son was put in jail for attempted robbery," she said with a catch in her voice.

"I'm so sorry you have to go through that, Mrs. Achey. Do you have other family close to you?"

"No, I live alone with my ten cats to keep me company. I love them more than my family, anyway!"

While I waited for her to make up her mind about a bath, I filled her pitcher with fresh water, fluffed her pillow, and tried to make her as comfortable as possible. Miss W, the instructor, aware that I was flustered and nervous, came to my rescue and together we bathed her and rubbed her back. Poor lady, she had to gasp for every breath she took, and I sure couldn't blame her for being uncooperative. I had a horrible feeling she was going to die. I'm so thankful she didn't die on my shift.

Two days later Riley and I were assigned to Katie, a senile 80-year-old lady who had suffered a stroke. We soon found out what a mess was ahead of us. Katie had come to the hospital from a nursing home with a horrible looking bedsore in her sacroiliac (tailbone) region. I kid you not! It was the size of a small dinner plate and had the putrid smell of – you guessed it – gangrene. She also had a bowel impaction. What a pitiful specimen of neglected humanity!

She was helpless, couldn't talk or move on her own, and breathed noisily through her dry, encrusted mouth. My stomach took a flip-flop and just about gave up its contents. Riley and I along with Miss W worked more than an hour to debride and clean the bedsore the best we could, give her an enema to relieve the bowel impaction, bathe her, give special mouth care, and make up her bed with clean linen. I couldn't eat dinner after doing all that. At that point, I really didn't care if I never ate another meal.

Another patient on my list was an elderly woman with her uterus hanging out. The doctor said she was too old to tolerate an operation, so he discharged her to go home later that day. She also had cancer of the liver that produced yellow jaundice. How sad. Her days are numbered, too.

Situations like these broke my heart! They fueled my desire to be a nurse more than ever so I could help people in their distress. That evening so many thoughts and feelings roiled around like a whirlpool in my mind.

February 20, 1951: *In nursing arts class today we did several things designed to help us empathize with our patients. We bandaged each* *other's eyes to better understand what it's like to be blind, we smeared a bit of Vaseline on our glasses to simulate blurred vision, we practiced feeding ourselves with our left hands to understand how it would be if our right arms were broken or paralyzed, we practiced using a cane and crutches to aid in walking, we put a big wad of cotton in our ears to simulate diminished hearing. My goal as a nurse is to be sensitive to what a person needs and be their eyes and ears. That exercise really focused on how to empathize with our patients who are deaf and blind and have other impairments.*

February 25, 1951: *Yesterday morning, I monitored three patients coming out from under ether anesthesia after surgery. The quickest way to get a patient to respond is to gently pinch the ears and neck. As the patient comes close to being responsive, he/she squirms and frowns when we do that.*

Mr. Shank had abdominal surgery. He is an obese person and as he thrashed around trying to turn on his side, he almost fell out of the narrow bed. It was up to me to keep him from doing such a drastic thing; I put up the bedrails and that helped a lot. He kept moaning for his wife, too.

I also monitored a post-operative patient who was getting an intravenous solution of glucose. It is much more interesting now that we are allowed to work with real patients.

February 26, 1951: Writing a long letter to Carl helped me calm down: *Dearest Carl, you better sit down to read this because I have lots to tell you. Let me introduce you to dear Patsy Witt. She is such a sweet patient who has pneumonia. After I put fresh linens on her bed and made her some toast and broth, she reached up and gave me two kisses – one on each cheek, great big smackers – I felt well paid. Then it seemed like everyone needed a bedpan at the same time. I never <u>ever</u> dreamed I would empty so many bedpans.*

At 7 p.m. we went off duty, terribly tired after four hours of patient care. If we're tired now, though, after only four hours, just think what it will be like when we work eight hour shifts! I dread the thought. It's a good kind of tiredness, though, and it is fun to work together as a team – we feel united with a sense of camaraderie. I was so weary I couldn't make myself go to prayer meeting at church this evening. Do you think God will forgive me? I know part of my fatigue is due to being on an emotional tension, striving to please patients and do work that's acceptable to my instructors.

Tomorrow morning I go back on duty at 7 a.m. so I must get some sleep. Three mornings this week I am scheduled for day duty. Oh, how my bones rebel against getting up at 5:55!! Ah, woe is me!

Guess what – Hennie just came and told me that Mrs. Achey died – (the lady with the hernia that I expected to die). She said the family was on their way to the hospital to take her home but by the time they got here, she was dead. Next time we go on duty, it will seem strange not to have crabby Mrs. Achey there.

Poor Katie died last Saturday. Her open oozing bedsore only got worse no matter what we did for her. The smell was nearly unbearable. I feel relieved and hope both Miss Katie and Mrs. Achey were ready for heaven. Poor souls, it was a blessing they could die. Neither of them would have had a good quality of life.

I finally have a weekend off and plan to spend it with Mollie and her family. It's been three weeks since I was there. I can't wait to get away from this busy, intense hospital routine. Maybe I'll get to see you this weekend? Gotta sign off and go nitey nite.   Love always, Minnie."

A hectic schedule begins to take a toll

Early morning ward assignments, heavy hospital duties, intense non-stop studies, and stiff final tests began to take their toll on all of us. Several classmates threatened to quit the program, but others talked them into staying and not giving up so easily. It would be demoralizing and discouraging if more students quit. This means we only had four options for venting our frustrations: complain about how tired we get, gripe about how hard we have to study, fret and fume about how unfair it is that we have to stay around for classes on our days off, cry and pull our hair when our one overnight weekend a month is canceled if we fail a test.

Learning how to balance our time off duty wasn't easy. We often had to cut a date short with a boyfriend or leave a concert early in order to meet curfew at midnight on Saturday or 10 p.m. on weeknights and Sunday.

During one of our infrequent times together, I told Carl that I must resolve to "hit the hay" in good time, especially if I was scheduled to work a day shift the next morning. Invariably I knew I would reap the consequences of a "blue Monday" if I didn't get to bed by 10 p.m. If I would snooze in class the gals teased me mercilessly. It was my own dumb fault, I knew.

Carl heartily agreed to honor my resolve. He didn't want to lose sleep, either. He said his professors can always tell by his bleary eyes when he burns the midnight oil too often. Since we didn't see each other more than every three or four weeks, it was hard to cut short our times together.

Chapter 5
Leisure Activities

Mixing play with work

In case there was any doubt about a balanced lifestyle for the students, such as "all work and no play" the reader can be assured there were occasional times of relaxation, parties, and fun, too. One of those times was a surprise party for my 20th birthday. Secretly, Mollie and her family invited several of my good friends from the college to come to a party at her home. She asked Carl to concoct a fictional reason to take me on a date so I would dress up a little bit. I was so surprised when my friends showed up instead. They gave me such useful and lovely gifts. Tears came to my eyes to think they would be so thoughtful. The group played games, pulled taffy, and had refreshments of sandwiches, corn curls, ice cream, and birthday cake. After everyone had gone home, Carl, Mollie, and I had fun cleaning up and washing the dishes together.

After the test in nursing arts class was over at noon one day, we were FREE for the weekend! I hurriedly packed my overnight bag, ate dinner, and caught a 2:15 p.m. bus to Mollie's home. Her mother had fixed a delicious supper that featured her specialty – a roasted stuffed pig's stomach – a traditional Pennsylvania German meal. The stuffing was spicier than stuffing used for turkey or chicken. I figured the extra spice was intended to cover up the flavor of the pig stomach. After she roasted it, she sliced it and served it with gravy. This was the first time I had ever eaten that delicacy. The name sounded awful but it tasted good, just different from anything I had ever eaten before. Can't say as I would want to eat it very often. Thankfully, it wasn't served all that often.

March 1, 1951: An excerpt from a letter to Carl describes extracurricular activities: *This is a peaceful and quiet Sunday afternoon – perfect for letter writing. Gracie and I are here in her room listening to Billy Graham on the radio and chewing on the big hard pretzels we get here. I could watch TV but there is absolutely nothing worthwhile on TV; it can go to the dogs, for all I care! I would much rather listen to good classical music on the radio.*

The church young people's party was a fun time last night. Gracie gave a reading and I played a piano solo. We played games, sang rollicking songs and, of course, ate lots of food.

Earl brought us back here at 12 midnight. Already, I broke my promise to make myself to go to bed early if I have early morning duty. Groan. Oh, well, we only live once, I tell myself.

March 2, 1951: *On Hennie's birthday we had a little snack – potato chips, doughnuts, candy, etc. Did I say a "little" snack? Is it any wonder that I feel fat? I was stuffed. My whole evening was wasted, but I didn't care. After being so serious on duty, we need to "pull out the stops" and have fun sometimes.*

Last night Mary and Jean were acting so silly. Mary doused Jean's head with Coca Cola. In return, Jean made tracks for the kitchen where she fetched a raw egg, came back and broke it over Mary's head! What a mess that made. Such is dorm life at good ole LGH.

If our work schedules allowed and the weather cooperated, Gracie and I walked the 16 blocks to the mission church for Sunday services and Wednesday prayer meetings. It was great exercise and took only 35 minutes. Pastor Walters gave such good sermons. Mrs. Walters often invited us for one of her super delicious Sunday dinners. We thoroughly enjoyed the splendid opportunities to get away from the suffocating hospital routine and socialize with a family.

Beginning long-awaited vacation

August 5, 1951: *I am happy, happy, happy – my long-awaited vacation begins. Hallelujah! I'll get to see my dearest Carl tomorrow. It seems like forever since we have had a chance for a good talk. My heart ached when I read his wonderful letter this week – to think we must be apart for two more long years - such a long time.*

He called to invite me to go deep sea fishing on Monday with the group from his church. I've never been out on the ocean before, so I readily accepted his invitation. He said there is room for me to ride in his car. What a grand way to start my vacation!

August 6, 1951 Sunday night, 11 p.m.: *My stuff is packed and ready to go. All I have to do now is figure out how to stay awake till 2 a.m. when the fishing party will pick me up. I'm scared to go to sleep even though I set two alarms. I'm afraid I'll turn it off and go back to sleep. My roommate and two others just came off evening duty, so I'll talk to them awhile. I'm so eager to go deep sea fishing for the first time I hardly know what to do! I'll tell you all about it after I get back tonight.*

When the first alarm sounded, I woke up, dressed, tip-toed to the front door in my stocking-feet, and clumsily dropped one of my shoes as I opened the heavy front door. I held my breath and listened intently, fully expecting Mrs. G, our housemother, to ask why I was trying to sneak out at such an ungodly hour. But not a soul stirred. So I went merrily on my way.

My job was to keep Carl awake since he said he hadn't had a chance to sleep first. Four others rode with us in his car. We followed Walter's car with three other people. We stopped to eat breakfast in a little podunk restaurant along the seashore that didn't give very good service.

At 7 a.m., we ambled down to the beach where our boat, *TAMBO III*, was moored. Our captain was a jolly old man who asked if Carl and I were married and teased us when we said we weren't.

I had been to the beach once before but had never gone deep sea fishing on the ocean. It was great sport swaying back and forth on the boat with the gently heaving waves – only sometimes it wasn't exactly gentle, No one got sick, however, and we had so much fun.

Carl landed the biggest fish of the whole catch of 26 fish. I caught only two or three, but what a thrill that was. The boat captain helped us clean them and put them on crushed ice. I also "caught" a painful sunburn on my face, arms, and legs.

After five hours of pure enjoyment pulling in fish, we devoured the brown-bag lunches we brought with us, and then headed home. We stopped at my dorm so I could pick up my overnight stuff for staying at Mollie's home. Three of my housemates – Heidi, Naomi and Jean – were lounging on the front porch, and they raved about my sunburn.

We drove to Kelly's home where we divided the fish. Each person took two big ones, and the drivers got two extra. I wish I had recorded the kinds of fish and how much they weighed.

We arrived at Carl's home about 6:30 p.m. only to find his mom had fixed guess what? fish for supper! I could hardly make myself look at a fish again. Sitting down to eat more fish was way over the top. I was exhausted beyond belief having had very little sleep for 36 hours, but oh so happy. It was worth every minute of it.

Reveling in romance

A few weeks later on a warm summer Sunday afternoon, Carl invited me go with him to a special picturesque spot along the wide swift-flowing Susquehanna River. He wanted to show me the spectacular view that he liked so much.

September 2, 1951: *As usual I picked up my journal when I got back. Often when I'm sleep-deprived, I'm not fit to be around anyone, but he is patient and puts up with my mercurial moods. Today I was very tired after being called out for surgery to help with a bleeding tonsillectomy at 4 a.m.*

I hadn't been awake very long and wasn't quite ready when Carl arrived to pick me up. We hadn't seen each other for several weeks. Being with him was like having a shot of vitamins in my arm – suddenly I wasn't tired anymore.

It turned out to be a splendid time together on this high, rugged, rocky cliff that hangs out over the wide, deep-flowing river. How simply wonderful to walk hand in hand and know everything was just "hunky-dory" between us. It was a gorgeous day with my sweetie.

The weather was perfect, sunny at first with not a cloud in the sky. Since we both love nature, we sat down to enjoy the sparkling view of the rushing river. Later we traipsed through the cool, wooded surroundings as we gathered firewood. We built a small bonfire to roast our hotdogs. Just as we devoured our last hotdog, the west wind suddenly and capriciously scattered our lunch stuff. The clouds quickly piled up gray and menacing in the western sky, and soon a cloudburst surprised us. We quickly gathered up our things, dashed to the car, crawled in, and listened to the rain pound around us for about fifteen minutes. The rain stopped almost as suddenly as it began. The sun came out, and a beautiful rainbow appeared in the east as the sun was setting – what a lovely end to the brief storm!

We lost track of the time and didn't notice how dark it was getting. We reluctantly cleaned up our campsite and headed home with the stars twinkling overhead in the inky sky.

I often had to finagle unique ways to maximize my time off duty when my crazy hospital work schedules interfered. I appreciated when good friends offered to pick me up from the bus station at odd times.

Many churches in the area were really big on revival meetings. Much of the year, a revival meeting was going on somewhere at one of the many area churches close by that we could attend if we wanted to hear preaching with altar calls. Carl was studying to be a minister so he frequently chose that kind of meeting for our dates. I grew up going to revival meetings, so I wasn't real thrilled about spending our limited time together at a revival meeting. But if that was how I could be with him, then that's where we would go. Having fun on our infrequent times together was more important to me than spiritual refreshment. I would much rather attend the college choir programs, young peoples' meetings at different churches, or spend time at the home of one of my "adopted" families. We did those things, too, on some dates.

I wrote in my journal after one of our outings: *This day has ended all too soon. Carl and I left the concert early because I had to be back by 10 p.m. Yes, I failed a test this week and lost my Saturday overnight privilege. Shoot the luck! Why in the world did I have to flunk that test? Oh well, that's life, I guess. Right now, I have half a notion to quit this place. Just a half, that is. Well, maybe not even that much. I get so eager to have a good time without having to meet a curfew.*

It was so wonderful to be with Carl, even for a short time. He made a special effort to pick me up. I know he will make a devoted husband some day. He's such a dear – I could just shout it to the world. We never get tired of talking. I just love him to my heart's content. Seems like our love grows stronger each time we're together. Blest be the tie that binds! Oh, oh, oh, I'm getting carried away – gotta get back to reality and go to bed. I must get up in time to work in the O.R. tomorrow. Duty calls.

I had a tendency to be depressed for several days after I visited my recently married friends in their homes. I was happy that they were married, but it was hard to see them living together in what appeared to be such perfect harmony and here I was slogging away for another two years. I thought how wonderful it must be to have all that close companionship and not need to say goodbye anymore. So I decided it was not in my best interest to visit them as often. Strange how relationships change after friends marry.

Enjoying Thanksgiving / Christmas, 1951

My schedule for this special holiday, Thanksgiving, was a split shift: work from 7 a.m. until 12 noon, off duty until 3:30 p.m., then go back to work until 7 p.m. Most of us did not like split shifts, but that's the way it was – one of those things that we had no control over and had to do it whether we liked it or not.

I had hoped to spend the holiday with Mollie or Carl's family, but with this crazy schedule I didn't see how that could happen. At 12:20 p.m., bless his heart, Carl picked me up and we drove the short distance to the home of his aunt and uncle. Carl's parents and sister were there, too. Oh my, what a sumptuous feast she had prepared: roast turkey, mashed potatoes, gravy, asparagus, creamed corn, piccalilli, cranberry sauce, celery, homemade butter, bread and jam, Jell-O with fruit and nuts, spicy pumpkin pie, all topped off with pink and white mints.

After stuffing myself, I felt like lying down and sleeping like a big fat pig would do. Instead, I had to go back to work. We played the piano and sang together before Carl brought me back to work. Even though it was brief, it was a great time to relax and visit with everyone.

December 11, 1951: *Several of us girls went to the Christmas program at the First Presbyterian church where the choir presented The Messiah. For 2 1/2 precious, fleeting hours I was so close to Heaven listening to that wonderful, soul-lifting music climaxed by the glorious Hallelujah Chorus. The soprano soloist was exceptional. My heart was strangely carried far above this trifling world, as though I had been given wings...great, white, silvery wings...and was hearing the trumpets of the angels as the orchestra accompanied the chorus. What will Heaven be like if earthly beings can render such music?*

It was a terrific jolt to come back down to earth as the last "Amen" died away in the echoes of the huge church sanctuary. Even after the benediction, my heart still thrilled and I tingled all over when I thought of that superb performance! Once again I must return to the mundane world and shoulder life's responsibilities, cares, problems and anxieties.

Another entry: *Oh, diary, I must tell you about the double date Jean and I had with our boyfriends. Eldon and Jean and Carl and I went to see the Bob Pierce movie "38th Parallel" at Youth for Christ. After the movie, we had a swell time of singing together at Jean's home. On the way back to the hospital, Eldon was driving along when a policeman stopped him and said, "Do you know why I stopped you?"*

"No, what did I do?" asked Eldon.

"You passed on the yellow line a mile back," the policeman informed him.

Eldon told him, "These lovely nurses have a curfew and I'm in a hurry to get them back to the hospital on time."

The policeman then graciously said, "OK, I won't give you a ticket this time. I know what that's like because my fiancé is a student nurse there, too. I have a warm place in my heart for nurses. Just be careful."
Wow, the fellows were sure glad they were with nurses that night!

On another Saturday night I wrote: *Mollie and I went to Youth for Christ to see another Bob Pierce film – "The Flame". It did something to me! Never have I been so moved to tears as when I saw the horrible conditions that exist in Korea. My emotions acted normally that night for a change. Usually I keep my feelings pent-up and shoved aside as a way of controlling them so they seldom have a chance to find expression in tears. Sometimes I wondered if I have any more tears. My unexpressed feelings create a painfully hard knot inside of me, an ache that leaves me exhausted and wretched. But that night I cried as I saw the skeletons of those poor innocent children, men, and women suffering from malnutrition who die seemingly for no reason.*

This has awakened my conscience about how I can sacrifice in small ways and pray more earnestly for the tremendous needs that were portrayed. I am glad I live in America. I won't take for granted the comforts and luxuries I'm privileged to enjoy. Millions are groping for the Light, the Flame of everlasting truth that could lead them into a glorious future! What a challenge to us as Christians to pray, go, and give.

Chapter 6
Giving Medications

Timid and fearful

Up until now I had practiced giving shots by injecting an orange, but one day in class I finally mustered the courage to plunge that hypodermic needle and sterile water into a real live person's arm. Why was I so timid and hesitant? I didn't want to hurt my friend Naomi, my classmate who had agreed to be my guinea pig. But that was part of what I had come here to learn, giving medications to help patients recover. I savored that big moment.

From my journal: *I shook nervously for at least two minutes as I decided how to make the final thrust of that glittering needle into a living person's arm! After it was all over, I chided myself for being so squeamish because there was absolutely nothing to it. She said she didn't even feel it. The sharp needle glided effortlessly into her fleshy upper arm as if it were soft butter – it was simple as falling off a log backwards. I had successfully leaped over another major hurdle.*

Boosting spirits

One balmy spring day, birds were singing, the breeze was balmy, and flowers were blooming. All this might have boosted my flagging spirits had I not been feeling so uptight and anxious about an anatomy and physiology test looming later that day. Even though I had studied till after midnight, I still did not feel prepared.

When I checked my mailbox, this upbeat letter was there from my sweetie:

Hello, sweet Marilyn! This lovely afternoon reminds me of when you were here in school last year. Remember when we walked the Minnemingo trail among the fragrant honeysuckle flowers and blooming magnolia trees? I sure wish we could do that again. I think I have spring fever these days.

I didn't go home last weekend because I caught this chest cold and didn't think it was wise to expose it to anyone else. I knew that if I went home I couldn't stay away from seeing you, and as usual we would have talked late. Now the edge cometh, where no man can write...Sincerely, Carl

I replied with a quick note:
Carl dearest, on a gorgeous spring day like this I also wish we could walk the woodsy forest trail where we could breathe in those heady fragrant perfumes and soak up nature's beauty. Here in the city we have cold, unresponsive streets, sidewalks and concrete walls all around us, with a few struggling patches of green grass and several scrubby evergreen bushes. It can be most depressing at times. Enjoy that natural beauty for me. I'll hang my close on this line for now. Love, M

Reading private mail

Those of us who lived in Foster House were very annoyed after we discovered our housemother was going through our drawers when she inspected our rooms each day. One of the girls even caught her reading her private letters. It really irritated us and stirred our righteous indignation to think of someone doing such a thing. I had suspected something was going on when I saw my drawer partially open one day. From then on mine went under lock and key. I had a notion to put a big sign in my drawer saying, "Hello, Miss Gore, will you kindly close the drawer, please? And don't ever open it again." Carol stormed into my room one evening in a total panic after finding her things disturbed. "Imagine such snoopervision!" she complained, stomping her foot down for emphasis. When I told Carol about my idea, we both laughed heartily.

Chapter 7
Dealing with Death and Dying

I was assigned to work on Men's Medical Ward for six weeks. What a drastic change from work with the women.

More journaling: *Oh, diary, I shall never be the same person as I was before. Today brought me closer to the angels in Heaven. I know they are rejoicing over one more devoted soul being ushered into the Kingdom forever.*

When I went to work this morning, I discovered my patient was one of the eminent missionaries to Africa. Mr. Elvin was admitted yesterday having suffered a heart attack and was not responding to stimuli. I did what I could to make him comfortable, but after hours of labored breathing in the big oxygen tent, he gave one deep sigh and then all was silent.

There was such a submissive and sweet look on his face as death set its impassive grip on his countenance. His wife's sorrowful sobbing was the only sound in the room as she faced the stark reality that her beloved companion was suddenly gone. I did what I could to comfort her. I told her that in my imagination, I visualized the angels coming down and bearing her devoted husband's soul up to realms ethereal. Pure imagination, I know, but I like to think about it that way. Through her tears she thanked me for being there with her.

This was my first real brush with death. I know it isn't wise to question God, but will somebody please explain to me just why such a useful servant – someone who was accomplishing so much for the Heavenly Kingdom – is suddenly stricken and laid to rest?

Dear God, why didn't you take old Mr. Craig, the man we admitted yesterday – dirty, decrepit, diseased, shoved around in the world, no one to care for him, dependent on society, no earthly place to call home except a disreputable hovel that wouldn't be fit for a dog to live in?

I'm reminded of the Bible verse, "God's ways are higher than our ways and His thoughts higher than our thoughts." I am more impressed than ever by the fact that this earthly life is like a puff of smoke compared to the endless length of all eternity.

I've been looking at life with different colored glasses since experiencing all the pain and suffering I see every day around here. Sometimes I think I'm wasting these three years in preparation for such a short life when there are so many desperate needs around me. I do know this is where I'm supposed to be right now, so I bend my efforts towards making the best use of all my opportunities while preparing for life itself.

This is turning out to be more of a philosophical discourse as I try to sort out how I feel about all this. After this experience with death, I must say, "How could I help but weep along with the family?" Touching scenes such as this one melt my nurse-heart very rapidly no matter how much I try to steel myself against the hard reality of pain and death.

My spiritual struggles and growing faith were being tested at several crucial points as I comforted families in pain when a loved one died. I did my best to ease intense physical and emotional suffering, minister to new mothers, care for newborns, and rejoice with patients who experienced hope and healing.

I wrote in my journal one evening as I was trying to relax: *Men's Medical Ward was such a difficult, busy place this morning. My assignment was five grumpy patients. I worked as hard and fast as I could to meet all the patients' demands before I was scheduled to go to pharmacology class at 10 a.m.*

The supervisor pranced around there acting like she owned the place. At one point she yelled at us, "Girls, get a little speed on you!" That really irritated and disgusted my buddies and me. I'd like to see her do everything for five difficult patients in three hours. It's at times like this I'm tempted to quit all this aggravation and hard work and go back home. Who needs these exasperating experiences that tend to create feelings of resentment? We're still just probies learning the ropes of this profession. We are bound to be slow and disorganized at times. After all that, I needed to do something to soothe my frazzled, frayed nerves and ruffled feathers so I went to play the piano and sing out my heart's cry.

One evening I added to my ever-expanding journal: *Dr. Hagan, an 82 year. old, nearly blind, retired Moravian minister, was my patient today. He had suffered a mild stroke and now has subacute bacterioendocarditis (a $20 name for heart disease, another one of my favorite long words). Says he taught homiletics in a seminary for 7 years. He could crack some of the funniest jokes. For instance, "Ever since woman was created after man, she's been after him ever since." I thought I would split laughing right there, but I managed to smile benignly and say, "Oh, I'll remember that joke. That's a good one, Dr. Hagan!" He's such a gentle man but at times he can really surprise us and crack us up royally.*

Another journal entry: *Mr. Turner must weigh 300 pounds, he is one big smelly mess, and I don't mean maybe. I nearly puked. Last night he asked for the "chamber" (bedpan) and when I came back to get it, he had thrown it on the floor and spilled the contents all over. Fortunately it was only urine this time, but I'll venture to say it's only a matter of time till it's more than that. He's just plain ornery. My initial reaction was to make him get out of bed and clean it up himself. But I restrained myself once again.*

Giving oral medications for the first time

Today was my first experience of actually giving oral medicines to patients on the ward – that's a big step in this process of learning. I've anticipated this day for a couple of months. What a responsibility it is, let me tell you truly. I was so nervous and afraid I would lose my focus and give the wrong medicine to somebody.

Well, it turns out that I did just that. I could have fallen through the floor from shame, embarrassment and, yes fear of dire consequences. Oh, how my face gets red to think I gave tincture of belladonna to Mr. Krane instead of Mr. Stabler. The dose was not critical so no harm done, thankfully. That just proves how easily mistakes can happen. I was surprised how sympathetic Miss B. was to me compared to how she has reacted to some of the other students when they blundered. At some point I am sure Mrs. K will call me in to her office and thoroughly rake me over the coals.

My journal two days later: *Oh dear! I knew it would happen... Mrs. K didn't waste any time calling me in to her office to confront me about giving that wrong medication. I was so scared I wished I could have fallen through the floor right there in her office. Would she send me packing out of here, I wondered? I shuddered as she scolded me thoroughly but she didn't say nasty things this time like she has sometimes. She did give me a stern warning just as if I'd committed a heinous crime. It's good, though, to be reminded that giving medicines is serious business and could turn out to be a disaster depending on what medicine was given and to whom. You can be sure I will be more careful to check the label three times like we've been instructed then read the patient's arm band carefully to avoid mistakes like that.*

Two days later, Miss B. again assigned me to pass pills and give injections. All went well this time. She said I had satisfactorily given medications, and supervision would no longer be required. What a sigh of relief went through my whole body; after that stunt I pulled the other day, I made sure to be much more vigilant. Live and learn. It seemed like I learned more by making mistakes than by doing everything right.

One of my letters to Carl graphically portrayed my mixed feelings: *Hi, Carl, Men's Medical is more interesting now that we are becoming better acquainted with the patients. You should have seen the filthy, unconscious bum that was brought in Friday night. He was probably homeless because he looked and smelled like he hadn't had a bath for a month. Hennie and I were assigned to give him a bed bath. We changed the water in the basin three times and he still wasn't clean. Our stomachs revolted at the sight of him but we dared not show it, just grimly went on with our task. He's still unconscious, by the way.*

Another patient showed his appreciation by insisting I take two of his Hershey candy bars. He was a kind old man and I enjoyed helping to make him more comfortable.

Carl, dear, here I am placidly blurting out stuff that probably bores you to death. Please forgive me for writing so much shop talk. Hopefully we'll get to see each other briefly when I come to the college activities this weekend. I'll try to get there in time to hear the chorus sing. I do miss that good choral singing. Wish I could stay for the panel discussion. I hate it that I have to leave early to get back by 10 p.m. Drats, that's life as a student nurse. I'm just glad I can come at all, though. Bye for now, M

Sharing the love of Christ

More journaling: *One morning while I was bathing Mr. Collins, he shared about how hopeless he feels when he listens to the world news.*

He said, "I've tried to live a Christian life, but sometimes I wonder if I were to be snuffed out like that (he snapped his fingers) I'm not so sure I'd be ready."

Since I had a few minutes to spare just then, I talked to him for about ten minutes and gave him some Scripture verses for later reference. I saw the grateful look in his eyes as he thanked me for helping him to see the "way" a little clearer. He asked me to pray for him, which I gladly consented to do. Each day I pray for wisdom for just the right thing to say to people when they initiate a conversation. I was glad to share my faith and hope with others.

When our final exam in nursing arts was over, I breathed a huge sigh of relief. I was so glad to have that behind me. Friday and Saturday were the finals in history of nursing and in medical science. Mrs. W. told us the results of our achievement test in microbiology and anatomy. I was shocked to learn that I was in the 99% group in micro and 89% group in anatomy. All that intense studying paid off, evidently.

Chapter 8
Women's Surgical Ward

More musings: *We started two new classes today – two more heavy-duty nursing books were thrown at us – medical nursing and surgical nursing. This is the way we swat 'em down one by one – subjects and finals, that is.*

My journal again came out from its hiding place: *Today didn't seem like Sunday at all. We are now working 8-hour shifts on the ward. We get really fatigued by the end of the shift. One's work is never done on a women's ward. Someone always needs something and the call bells ring constantly.*

You should see Women's Surgical – it's a riot at times. One of the patients is a tiny 80 year old woman who weighs only 68 lbs. I can lift her into and out of bed with no trouble. The other day she found out I was from another state.

"Well, how did you get here?" she asked in her squeaky, trembling voice. She had a twinkle in her eye and a mischievous grin on her wrinkled face. After a minute she exclaimed, "Oh, I know – I'll bet you have a boyfriend here."

I had to laugh at her innocent supposition and responded with, "Mrs. Berman, whatever gave you such an idea?"

Then she giggled self-consciously and said, "Oh, I just know how those things go. You see, I was your age once upon a time."

Another lady presented nursing staff with a big box of Hershey candy bars. She wants to make sure we stay nice and plump, I think. At this rate, we surely will. I think that we run it off in the course of a day's work, though.

One day the police brought a woman in whose husband had beaten her until she was terribly bruised, bleeding, had a broken arm, and was unconscious from a concussion. He had threatened to kill her. The cops told us that he had escaped from jail the day before and was still on the run. That really shook up my teammates and me. We never knew from one minute to the next what ugly situations we would have to deal with next. We had to stay as calm and collected as possible.

A judge's restraining order was in place so the doctor wrote an order for us to call the police if her husband attempted to come up on the ward. When the other patients on the ward heard the ruckus and saw the police roaming around, they were so scared they hunkered down in their beds and pulled their bedsheets up over their faces. Later that evening we were told the police caught the man and locked him up again.

Lo and behold the next day they informed us that he managed to escape again, so we still had to watch out for a maniac. He must have been one savvy prisoner. What was the matter with those guards at the jail, anyway? Nothing more ever happened, thankfully, and the patient was later discharged to a women's safe house.

My journal further describes our fast-paced work: *What a hairy day this has been! I'm at my wit's end physically and emotionally tonight. After eight hours on Women's Surgical, I feel as tired as if I had been digging a six foot ditch all day. That ward is a riot! Women are much harder to please than men are. Four of us probies had to figure out how to manage our patient assignments to get everything done before shift change.*

It was obvious that Mrs. Plast was very weak, her fingernails and lips were turning blue; she was vomiting and groaning. We knew she wouldn't last long. Sure enough, about 9:15 she breathed her last. Poor soul, she had a horrible death. Her common law husband took it very hard.

The graduate nurse on duty helped me get her body ready for the undertaker to pick up. I closed her glassy eyes, tied up her jaws, tied her hands and feet together, packed her body cavities with wads of cotton, put a diaper on her, and then wrapped her in the sheet-shroud. Taking care of a dead person isn't as bad as I thought it would be. With two of us working together, it went easier than I expected. I went off duty feeling wiser, more mature, and also keenly aware of the futility of a life such as she must have lived. Only God is her judge.

We raced around like mad for the next few hours. Two patients required constant attention when they went into shock on their return from surgery. Emergencies make us think fast and challenge us to do our very best nursing. Five patients needed to be prepped for tomorrow's surgeries. We admitted four new patients among other countless tasks to do. If we organize our work right, it can be satisfying. Eventually, when things simmer down again, we end up incredibly tired with our heads spinning wildly.

Imagine, after all that activity, when my eight-hour shift was over I dashed to my room, doffed my uniform, took a quick shower, and primped a bit. Carl picked me up right on time, and away we went to our good friend's wedding. You would never have known I had met life and death situations an hour before. I guess that's what it means to be a quick change artist. I almost feel like an elastic band being pulled in two different directions.

Diary, the work part doesn't bother me so much but what gets on my nerves is when the instructor tells me to do something, then in the middle of doing that, the head nurse comes and says, "Do this." When "this" is done, that first job isn't finished on time and then the instructor jumps on me for not having "that" job done. That riles me up inside something awful. Maybe they want to test me and see how I react to confusing orders. Outwardly, I grin and sweetly say, "Yes, Miss M," but inwardly I grit my teeth and say, "GRRR!" I just have to overlook things like this and move on, I guess. Give me clear instructions, not confusing orders, and I'll do my best work.

During my six week tour of duty on Women's Surgical Ward, I cared for many types of patients: fractured legs and arms, appendectomies, colostomies, spinal surgery, hysterectomies, just to name a few. There was never a dull moment as we dashed around madly doing surgical preps and giving pain medications to keep them comfortable.

Part Two

Six Months as a Junior Student

Chapter 9
Our Capping Ceremony

March 13, 1951: *Whoopee! A very special occasion happened today – we completed our six months of probation. We thought this day would never come. Our hearts palpitated with pleasure to know we had come this far in our nursing career. Six months ago we weren't sure if we'd make it to this point.*

A couple of days before the ceremony, just for fun, I went to Gracie's room and tried on one of her student caps to see what it felt like to wear that white, starched, bulbous cap perched perilously on my head and fastened to my hair with bobby pins. It felt strange but oddly satisfying as I anticipated wearing it on duty with my uniform.

What a riotous frenzy on second floor that evening as eight of us vied for the bathroom to prepare for the big event. We were each issued the starched white bibs for our blue and white striped uniforms finally. Each bib has the word "Miss" and the student's last name embroidered on the upper left. Mine says "Miss Minter." We helped each other fasten our stiff pristine white bibs to our white aprons with pearl button studs. The straps had to be crossed just right in the back. We lined up in the classroom where Mrs. K. gave us precise instructions and meticulously inspected each one of her girls individually. She looked us up and down from head to toe to make sure everything was in order. That took a chunk of time with 51 of us.

We all piled on the waiting bus at 7:50 p.m. Soon we were on our merry way to Franklin & Marshall College where the capping ceremony was to be held in the auditorium. When we were given the signal, 51 soon-to-be juniors in our starched uniforms marched jauntily down the aisle to take our seats. Draped over our left arms were the navy blue wool capes with bright red lining and "LGH" embroidered in gold letters along the stand-up collars. Those toasty warm soft capes over our uniforms protected us on cold windy days when we walked outside from building to building.

After listening to an excellent address by Dr. B. we paraded on stage to receive our coveted student caps as our names were called. I feared

I would do something dumb when I walked across the stage, like stumble up the steps or trip over something on the platform. Thankfully that didn't happen.

Mrs. K. beamed one of her infrequent broad smiles as she carefully pinned my cap to my dark brown hair. I thought about the times when I feared I'd never make it to this point of having that symbol of hard-earned achievement – a white cap, sitting precariously on top of my head. What a fantastic, heart-fluttering feeling! I don't think I've ever been more elated in my life. If I can make it through these first difficult six months, I am quite sure I can take whatever comes during the next 2 ½ years.

When the ceremony was over, we lined up at the back of the auditorium to greet our friends and loved ones as they came to congratulate us. Carl was there along with his mother, sister, and several of my college friends. After saying goodbye to our well-wishers, we boarded the bus and whizzed back to the dorm where a BIG party was going on. Such a riotous celebration! I don't think I can sleep tonight – I'm too wound up and excited. Tomorrow is my day off so I can sleep in – Goody!

Oh yes, Darcy hoped we would be allowed a midnight curfew so she asked Mrs. K. what time we must be in our rooms tonight. Mrs. K. frowned at her and retorted in her usual semi-sarcastic tone of voice, "Well, it seems as though you would want to go straight to your rooms and meditate for the next two and a half years on what you just heard tonight. Of course, you must be in by 10."

Sooo… that settled that.

"Who wants to meditate, anyway?" I said with an edge of desperation in my voice. "I feel like doing something wild and crazy!"
Jean retorted, "Darn it, the chances of that happening around here are next to none! I dare any of us to try."

Not all of our classmates persevered to the bitter end of the probation period. It is amazing that only four dropped out along the way. One got sick, two flunked out, and one quit because it leaked out that she was secretly married.

Celebrating caps leads to challenges

It took some time to get used to the idea that we were no longer on probation. We were junior nursing students instantaneously, infused with added self-confidence at the flick of a white cap pinned on our heads. There was a certain settled feeling about that. Anyone else had to experience it to know what that felt like. Both students and graduate nurses wore their caps with pride as symbols of achievement.

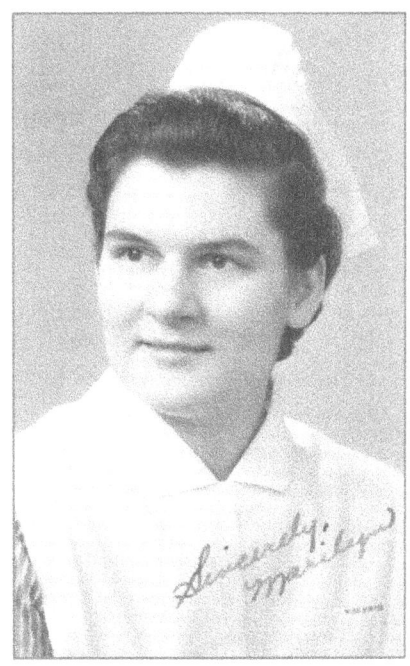

In another six months we would be intermediate students, and a year after that we would be senior students. Each new level would carry with it added serious responsibilities. Almost before we knew it, three years would pass and we would be graduate nurses ready to conquer the world!

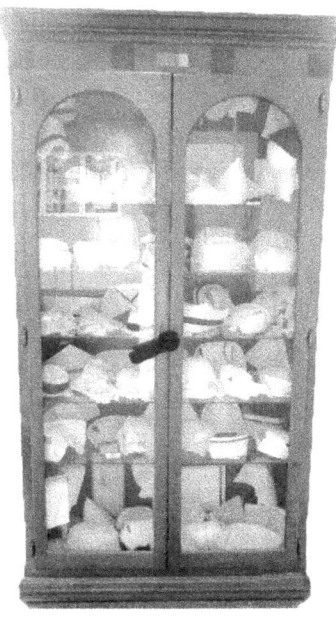

At that time each hospital-based diploma nursing program had a distinctive style of cap for their graduate nurses. By 1970, the long-standing practice of nurses wearing white caps had dwindled to almost nothing. The demise of the cap loosely coincided with men coming into the profession in the seventies. The male nurses objected to wearing caps, and female nurses were glad for the excuse not to wear one. The fact was that in performing certain nursing procedures, the cap was definitely a hindrance.

Sometimes it either fell off or was knocked off in the process (www.nursinghistory.org/nursing-cap-collection).

Currently wearing a white cap and white uniform is optional in some hospitals. They do add a touch of dignity and professionalism, in my opinion. I have heard doctors and patients both express frustration when they can't tell the difference between the graduate nurse and the cleaning woman down the hall since both wear shapeless scrubs and have no caps ("Where did the nurse's cap go," www.medscape.com/viewarticle/741581).

Back to the grind

In April 1951, spring weather brought trees and grasses back to life. Balmy breezes warmed the cold earth. Stirring mysteriously in my heart were memories of the woodsy trail at the college where Carl and I had walked hand in hand. Spring fever returned in full force. Reality, though, stared me in the face. Studies piled up at the end of the spring semester.

It was torture trying to study for that dreadful pharmacology final. When that was over, I could have gone out and turned a somersault, done a handspring, whatever. That was so nerve wracking. I could only hope I would pass the dumb thing.

Term papers were due. Final tests weighed us down and robbed us of precious sleep. We neared exhaustion from so much classwork, studies, and hospital duty combined in a 24-hour period. Everyone rejoiced at the prospect that classes were scheduled to end the middle of June. We would have two whole months without classes, term papers, and finals until the first of September. We could then work with patients and not be weighed down with studies, too. That thought was almost too good to be true.

Chapter 10
Operating Room Experience

Navigating the operating room

April 12, 1951 A quick entry in my journal: *In 3 more days, I rotate to the operating room for eight weeks. Now that scares me a whole bunch. We have so much homework to study in the operating room techniques class. I feel nervous already since I know that Miss Nord, one of the supervisors, is super particular about sterile technique. In an operating room that's SO important. I'm sure I'll learn one way or another – probably by making lots of dumb mistakes.*

The middle of April, six of my classmates and I began our operating room (O.R.) rotation together. We were plagued with misgivings and nervous tension about how we would handle this most exacting part of our experience. This was even more anxiety-producing than giving those first medications.

After a few days in the O.R., my long weekly letters to Carl reflected a lot of optimism:

Things here are really going great. I couldn't wish for it to be any better. I just love the O.R. It really surprises me at how super the staff has been to us. It makes it easier to absorb the huge amount of information that has been given to us. Miss A is the big-shot supervisor up there, and these last few days she explained everything so thoroughly. I needn't have worried as much as I did. Yesterday I stood back and observed an operation, but today I actually scrubbed in for an operation just like the surgeons have to do.

Here's what we do to get hands and arms as sterile as possible: using antiseptic soap, I scrub both hands and arms up to my elbow and around each finger with a stiff brush for 8 minutes. I dry them off with a sterile towel. Then I dip them in a basin with mercuric chloride and in another basin with alcohol. I use another sterile towel to dry my arms and hands.

The canopy (instrument) nurse must also go through this sterilizing ritual. The circulating nurse doesn't have to do that. What she does is hold a sterile gown, mask, and gloves for me to put on in a special way, and then I am considered sterile enough to assist the doctor with the surgery. We must go through this entire procedure between each operation so our skin becomes dry and scaly, or even raw sometimes.

When I was entirely "sterile," Miss A. told me to stand by the doctor and hand him the right instruments. That was awesome to hold the retractors that keep the incision open. Doctor A. explained everything clearly as he went along. Now the trick is to retain all that knowledge as fast as I get it. Tomorrow I will be instrument (canopy) nurse. That involves placing all the instruments and equipment on a tray in the exact order the surgeon needs them for that day's surgeries. It's quite a skill in itself to learn how to set that up.

The surgeries I have observed and assisted with so far have been two cholecystectomies (removal of gallbladder), tubal ligation, a hip replacement, and a semi-lunar cartilage removal.

Today we had two stat (emergency) surgeries. A lady required a Cesarean section and gave birth to a bouncing baby boy. A 20-year-old man needed his inflamed appendix removed.

On weekends we clean, clean, and clean some more. Everything cleanable is wiped down with antiseptic, including the tiled walls, leaving the place gleaming and immaculate. When we're done, I like that antiseptic squeaky-clean feeling.

Next week for a few days, I will work in the EENT OR. In other words, anything that has to do with surgery on ears, eyes, noses, and throats. This is where we do tonsillectomies, cataract removals, and mastoidectomies. I must close for now. Love, Marilyn

Once I got the hang of things, I could set up the canopy and instruments in 15 minutes. One time I had to stand there for three long hours assisting Dr. A. for two complicated spinal operations, both on the lower vertebrae. The doctor, surgical, and canopy nurses needed to have sturdy bladders because there was no time to take a potty break.

Wow, I was dead on my feet by the time that was over. My back ached terribly. I was ready for him to do surgery on my back to relieve the pain.

April 23, 1951: *In the afternoon, I assisted Dr. H. with an abdominal hysterectomy and an appendectomy. He is quite an interesting guy to talk to. We got into a discussion of television and religion while he was suturing the incision. He's done so many surgeries he can almost suture them with his eyes shut, I believe.*

Gracie and I ate supper in the cafeteria. but for some strange reason we couldn't stand to even look at the red beets and cherry crisp that were served. They looked too much like that bloody, yucky procedure we just finished. After supper, we walked outside to fill our lungs with fresh, cooler air. It felt good to get away from the non-air conditioned surgery even though the outside air was very humid.

Air conditioning is non-existent anywhere in the hospital. With no central air circulating, it gets so hot in the O.R. Standing at the canopy all decked out with that heavy paraphernalia, I could feel the perspiration trickle down my back, face, and neck. Since I had on sterile gloves I couldn't wipe it off, so I practically floated away – not literally, of course. I wouldn't exaggerate, now, would I? After the appendectomy, we gladly pulled off our perspiration-soaked gowns, gloves and face masks.

(I had always liked to tease by exaggeration and use of hyperbole, but Carl didn't like it when I did that. He always interpreted things so very literally. He told me one time he thought that exaggeration was next thing to telling a lie. Oh my! Did I have to try harder not to tease or exaggerate, or could I just be me?)

After all the surgeries were over for the day, we cleaned shelves and walls. It was a wonder the paint didn't come off of everything as often as we scrubbed the walls and equipment. Sterility was priority, though. "Cleanliness is next to Godliness," the Bible says. What a life of sterility this is.

One weekend we had Open House at the hospital, including the surgical suites. Miss A. had us practically turn everything upside down and inside out in the two operating rooms in an effort to have it meticulously clean. I'm sure we could have eaten food off the floor, too.

My initial optimism and enjoyment of the O.R. came to an abrupt end one day. I was doing so well in the O.R. until I made a dumb mistake. Inadvertently, I put an unsterile retractor in a sterile basin. Miss A. chewed me out good, said she lost confidence in me so I had to redeem myself by starting all over and getting everything sterile again.

Another goofy thing I did that was especially frustrating - I put surgical gloves in one autoclave and two flasks of water in another one to sterilize them. The gloves were to be autoclaved a half hour and water for an hour, but I failed to mark on the autoclave which was which. As a result, the gloves were done an hour and the flasks of water a half hour. I panicked. Oh dear, what's going to happen to me? I'll probably be banished and given menial tasks to do. No harm was done, though, thankfully.

Unfortunately, I did dumb stuff like that every now and then and wondered if I would ever learn. My supervisor was provoked and scolded me for lack of attention to detail. After that happened, I went to my room and bawled like a baby out of pure frustration.

Having to be so particular and meet such high standards of sterility could be nerve-wracking over time, to say the least. I learned something about myself through all this, though. Being precise 100 percent of the time is not one of my strengths. I'm more of a big picture person rather than a detail person. The world needed my kind of a person too, I concluded.

May 9, 1951: *Now a load is off my chest. My drug chart for pharmacology is finished. I didn't have to go on duty till 10 this morning, so it was heavenly to sleep in a bit longer.*

Drats! I flunked that dumb materia medica test yesterday. Oh dear! I must do better in that stuff because I'm close to flunking the course.

Between all the demanding O.R. stuff, plus classes and tests it's all getting on my nerves. I feel like screaming! [Materia Medica is a branch of medical science that deals with the sources, nature, properties, and preparation of drugs] *It seemed like we were having major tests at least three times a week. I better study for the big test coming up tomorrow. I'll be so glad when classes are over in another month.*

Miss A. is on vacation, and the atmosphere has been very tense in the O.R. The two graduate nurses are difficult to get along with. Miss N. and Miss K. are very critical and irritable lately for some reason – probably because Miss A. isn't here to smooth things over. As it turns out, they each struggle to be the boss. They give us juniors confusing orders and fly off the handle at every minor discrepancy in protocol. Let's hope next week is better than this one because it is really nerve-wracking. We'll all be glad when Miss A. is back next week.

May 11, 1951: *I'm so glad today is over. Miss N. has been giving us juniors a hard time. She expects us to know more than we do so we end up feeling like fools if we don't know it.*

The supervisor returns

May 14, 1951: *This has been a momentous day – what a change this O.R. underwent now that Miss A. is back from vacation. You'd never know it was the same place! The tension was so thick last week we could cut it with a knife. The graduates barked at each other and also bossed us students around mercilessly. Everything is running smooth as silk now.*

This is my 6th week here in the O.R., with only two more weeks to go. Several of us got together tonight and studied like fury for that dreadful nervous system test tomorrow.

Some of the results of our final tests came in: my grades were 89 in nutrition, 88 in nervous system, and 83 in circulatory system. Not too bad, but I wished it would have been better. I blamed my mediocre grades on sleep deprivation, extreme fatigue, and long working hours in addition to classes and tests. There was never any let-up in the pressure.

Each of us O.R. nurses took our turn being on call for 24 hours. Emergency (stat) surgeries weren't as exciting as I thought they would be. I had to crawl out of bed at unearthly hours and stand bleary-eyed beside the surgeon. My tired brain tried to remember which instrument the doctor would demand next. One time I ended up feeling foolish after I unintentionally handed Dr. P. the wrong forceps. His short temper flared, and he forcefully threw the instrument against the wall and shouted a swear word. Thankfully I had the correct forceps I could hand him, and that calmed him down a bit.

One night when Shirley and I were on call in the O.R., we admitted two emergency surgeries, an appendectomy, and a bowel obstruction that required a blood transfusion and a colostomy. It was 3 a.m. when we finished cleaning everything and could settle ourselves in bed again. Next day we felt so crabby and dragged around to classes with dark circles under our eyes.

May 20, 1951: *All we did today was clean, clean and clean some more – shelves, walls, everything. What a job. Miss A. was on duty with us and we managed to have fun doing a less than desirable task. Working all day Sunday really kills the spirit in me. If I can't go to church it seems like the whole week can go wrong.*

May 28, 1951 This entry in my journal reflected my impatience for nursing school to end: *The baccalaureate service for the senior class was held at Grace Lutheran Church. They looked so beautiful in their all-white uniforms and graduate caps. Oh, if only I could be in their shoes and be this near to the end.*

Two nights later the graduation ceremony was held at the same place. It thrilled all of us to watch Mrs. K. hand the seniors their hard-earned diplomas. Just think, 2 years from now it will be us/me. What a joyous day that will be.

I liked being the O.R. circulating nurse once I knew more of what to do and less precision was necessary. At first it was pretty rough and nerve-wracking until I caught on to all that was involved. The circulating nurse assisted both the surgeon and the scrub-in nurse by doing errands that didn't require wearing a sterile gown and mask. Sometimes she used a towel to wipe the perspiration from our foreheads so it wouldn't drip into the surgical site. Oh my, that would be disastrous.

Miss N. was a fuss-button much of the time which could really get on my nerves if I let it. Sometimes I just had to agree with her and then go on about my business.

May 30, 1951: *Again I sit with pen in hand to chat with you and relate the day's experiences. They haven't been very exciting because there were no scheduled surgeries over the Memorial Day holiday. We spent most of the time doing grunt work: cleaned shelves, made sponges, wrapped sponges, rolled gauze or sheet bandages, etc.*

Tonight I was on call when Jane, one of our classmates, had to have a stat appendectomy at 1:00 a.m. I scrubbed in as the assistant to Dr. H., the surgeon. Ruthie did a good job as my circulating nurse. Mary was my instrument/canopy nurse.

June 2, 1951: *By 10 a.m. I was again on duty and worked straight through till 7 p.m. We had very little to do besides cleaning, but Miss K. was too stingy to let us off early. Since I was on call for the next 24 hours, I didn't really mind too much.*

The crowning moment finally arrived. I completed my rotation in the O.R. Eight weeks earlier I started out with such a positive spirit. But as I got further into the nitty gritty details, it became more and more burdensome. Overall, it was a good learning experience. I decided that I was not cut out to be a surgical nurse, though.

June 3, 1951: *Carl surprised me by suggesting that we go on a picnic in the park after I got off duty. What a perfectly delightful way to celebrate the end of my eight week rotation in the operating room. We hadn't had any stat surgeries the night before, so I wasn't totally exhausted or grouchy like I've been sometimes after losing sleep.*

Zooming heat index

As summer rolled around, the humidity and heat index zoomed higher and higher and it became harder to concentrate on working eight hour shifts caring for patients. There was no central air anywhere in the dorms or the hospital rooms. It was difficult to sleep at night, too. Taking a shower/bath left a person still feeling hot and sticky, so no relief there.

June 5, 1951: *This evening after getting off duty, several of us who lived in Bowen House were sitting out on the porch chairs hoping to cool off in the early evening breezes. We hadn't yet changed into street clothes and were still wearing our student uniforms. Soon a strange man, about 40-years-old, walked right up to the bottom of the porch steps, looked at us quizzically, and immediately started talking to us:*

"Nurses' uniforms always do something to me. They turn me on," he said. "My first love was a nurse when I was 13 years old!"

We just sat there without responding. He went on to tell us intimate details about himself. Said he has had multiple sclerosis for 10 years and now gets some kind of shots for it. He said the brain disease had killed him sexually, but it waited long enough for him and his wife to have two children. He prattled on and on about his job and his extramarital love affair. We were too stunned to say anything and found it hard not to laugh in his face.

He stopped jabbering only after Shawna announced at 8 p.m. that she had to study for a test. The rest of us heaved big sighs of relief as we followed her into the house. He wandered on down the street whistling a jaunty tune. He never did tell us his name, and we didn't ask.

When he was out of earshot, Jean said with an edge of disgust in her voice, "Honestly, you could sure tell he has something wrong with him besides a muscle disease. His brain needs an overhaul, too." Good riddance.

Chapter 11
Men's Medical Ward / Evening Duty

Dealing with men, old and young

In June, Naomi and I were assigned for a nine week stretch to Men's Medical Ward where there were mostly decrepit, elderly men. After spending eight weeks in the operating room, it took me awhile to refresh my memory about what to do on a medical ward again. The routine gradually came back to me. It was a whole different kind of nursing with quite a conglomeration of patients. Here's a sampling.

June 6, 1951: *Mr. Witt has multiple sclerosis and is a pathetic sight. His muscles have atrophied to the point that he can't do much of anything for himself.*

Mr. G. is really a mess – talks the most nonsense you ever heard. His doctor can't decide what is wrong with him. In my opinion, he's just mentally off balance, that's all.

Mr. Lemm is in for a lot of tests and is a pleasant old man who loves to sing "La Dolce Vita" (The Sweet Life) at the top of his tenor voice. Says he used to sing in the opera. The other patients don't seem to mind. He doesn't give us any trouble.

Mr. Wise is also an ideal patient, a cooperative, pleasant personality, a lot of fun to talk to, and seems to be more cultured. He has a bleeding peptic ulcer. We treat it with two ounces of pure cream every two hours to coat his stomach lining, neutralize his stomach acids, and allow his ulcer to heal.

Mr. Seich is quiet and well-mannered. He is troubled with frequent nose bleeds and may need surgery. He has a heavy German accent and is hard to understand sometimes.

Mr. Axe is very nice. In fact, he's one of my favorites. He had a gastrostomy (stomach operation) today for a duodenal ulcer.

Jack Eisen, in the bed next to Mr. Axe, was admitted today. He is a good-looking, likeable fellow recently released from a three year prison sentence for attempted armed robbery. Last night about midnight, he and two other fellows led the police on a merry chase at 100 miles an hour down through town and out in the country. We were told they flattened 3 gas tanks and their car overturned at a sharp curve. Jack escaped with only a broken hand, head lacerations, and a back sprain. He can be thankful it wasn't worse. Guess God wants him to have another chance.

He's 25 years old and, in my estimation, he seems like too nice a guy to be an ex-convict. I don't know how the other two fellows survived. They were taken to another hospital. Later that evening, after I had settled all my patients for the night, Jack approached the nurses' station where I was charting.

I chided him gently, "Jack, why aren't you in bed? You need your beauty sleep."

He replied in his deep husky voice, "I couldn't sleep, so I thought I'd come and talk to you for a while."

I listened while he talked frankly about his difficulties: "I got in with the wrong crowd several years ago and, even though I only drove the get-away vehicle, I was accused of attempted bank robbery and spent thirty six months in prison. It's a long story."

I made a comment on how God can help us in our everyday life if we let him.

"Where do you go to church?" he asked.

When I told him he said, "Don't be surprised if I show up there some Sunday. When I was a kid my grandma took me to church. I learned that God loves me, but I haven't gone to church for a long time…maybe I will start again."

"Why did you stop going to church?" I asked.

"I really don't have a good reason why I quit going to church. I want to do what's right, but I'm not disciplined enough to follow through. What I really want now is to finally settle down, be serious and get married."

He went back to bed, and I continued on with my charting. His openness to God's love really touched me.

After our visit I had a lot of mixed feelings. This was way out of my comfort zone, but I admit I was a bit flattered that he wanted to talk to me. Did I do the right thing by talking to him? Did he think I was flirting with him? Was he flirting with me? He'll probably be discharged tomorrow, so he won't bother me from now on.

The next evening, I was alone at the charting desk again. I was so surprised when Jack sauntered jauntily down the hall during visiting hours. As he passed the nurses station, he told me he had been discharged home earlier in the day but came back to visit his friend Mr. Axe. After they visited a few minutes, he came back to the nurses' station, winked at me, and said playfully, "I didn't only come to see Mr. Axe. I came to see you."

He continued, "I can't sleep because every time I turn over I see your face in front of me, and I think of the things you've been telling me. My family is at home playing cards and drinking beer. I'd rather be up here talking to you."

I was really flabbergasted; what was I supposed to say? I really wanted this conversation to end. This was getting out of control. I decided to laugh it off. "Oh, you're just kidding me,"

He emphatically said, "Believe me, I am really serious."

By the tone of his voice, I believed him, but I informed him as clearly as I knew how, "I am already in a serious relationship and am not interested in anyone else."

That seemed to stop him in his tracks, but he hung around until I finished charting and gave report to the night nurse. Then he asked if he could walk me to my residence. When we said goodnight, I had a niggling feeling he was in love with me. He seemed like a nice fellow, but I didn't want him hanging around.

I was shocked again when I got a letter from Jack a few days later! Honestly, what was I supposed to do? He said he still liked me an awful lot and wanted to write to me. I ignored his letter and never saw him again after that. I often wondered what happened to him. I am still naïve about male-female relationships, so it was a teachable moment for me to be aware of how easy it was to get too involved with a patient, especially a charming, good-looking man.

June 10, 1951: *Here's a current sampling of Men's Medical Ward patients with multiple problems: senility, cardiac ailments, stomach ulcers, pneumonia, and lots more. We sure do have a mixture of patients now.*

Mr. Jasik keeps talking about his beautiful teeth. Mr. Swope tells us that he is 73 and says his father is 41. Now just how can that be?

I was changing Dr. Yeager's sheets, and what do you think he did when I leaned down to tie his gown and fluff his pillow? Grabbed me around the neck and kissed me! I nearly laughed in his face. He says I'm the best nurse of them all. He probably tells all his nurses that.

Mr. Snyder informs me about what love is after marriage and teased me about walking down the street with a baby carriage.

Working eight hours on the wards in the summer heat and humidity with no air conditioning anywhere was like enduring punishment. Some days were so sultry and hot we just barely slogged through a shift. Fighting the heat left us more fatigued by the time we went off duty. The patients minded the heat, too. Many times there wasn't a breath of air moving. Sometimes if we were not very busy, it was hard to keep our minds off of being hot. What a relief to go back to our rooms, take a bath, and perhaps congregate out on the front porch hoping to catch a vagrant breeze as we re-hashed the day's or evening's activities. Or maybe someone would walk by and tell us his/her life story like that guy did one time. The spice of life made life interesting. We never knew what to expect next.

June 12, 1951: *It seemed like everything that could go wrong did go wrong on this evening shift. First of all, as I went to give Mr. Jacobs an injection, the needle bent at a perfect right angle! Wow, I was jarred and so was he. He wasn't real happy about having to be stuck twice.*

I said to him, "I'm so sorry, Mr. J. I must go back and get another syringe and needle. I apologize for having to stab you again." Bless his heart, he didn't complain.

By 10 p.m. we had all 25 patients settled in their beds and everything was calm and peaceful. After I dimmed the lights, Mr. Moore rang his bell and asked me to empty his urinal. What did I do? Accidentally tipped it the wrong way and urine spilled all over his bed and on to the floor. What a mess to clean up. My nickname should be "Messie" instead of "Minnie."

Then about 10:30, just when I thought I had each one relaxed, back-rubbed, quieted down, and asleep, Mr. Shane dropped his bedpan on the floor. What a racket and another big mess. The terrible noise was like a gun shot in the night that woke everybody up again. Before they could go back to sleep, everyone needed something – a drink of water or a urinal. Then another round of charting was necessary. Needless to say, it was near midnight when I went off duty.

After spending all that energy, Sherrie and I were so tired we could hardly drag ourselves up the steps to our rooms. No one knows or cares or would believe how tired we become by running our poor old legs off for eight hours on the ward. The last thing I felt like doing was study for the gastrointestinal final tomorrow. But like it or not, I must do it.

Just think, tomorrow is the last class and the last test until September. Yippee! Finally our tired brains can take a much-needed rest. What a gloriously thrilling thought. It will seem like we've been released out of prison.

Gracie finishes her three-month psychiatric rotation in Philadelphia next week. I've missed her so much and can hardly wait for her to come back so we can do things together. She will work here until she is finished with the program in September. My roommate, Naomi, isn't as eager to go places and do things with me as Gracie is. Mollie has a whole different schedule, but she and I go places together as often as we can.

June 13, 1951: *Confession time: I started to study last night, but my head drooped lower and lower until it rested on the table. Before I knew it, I was fast asleep. One of the girls woke me up an hour later with no studying done. I was too tired to do more. My grades have been As and Bs up to now, so I told myself I would wing it on this one. Then I hopped into bed. Aah, blessed rest.*

Our final exam over the gastrointestinal system was terribly difficult today. What a bummer. But hallelujah, that marks the end of our classes for the summer – from now on till September we are FREE. I also have two whole days off for the first time. I'm not sure how to handle all that! I've become so used to classes and curfews for the last nine months.

Classes and tests finally ended for the summer, and we were free to come and go as we pleased during our times off duty. No more studies until September. Feature that! We were even granted the privilege of staying out an extra half hour, until 10:30, every night. Small wonders never cease!

Chapter 12
Personal Sickness, Moving and Vacation

Ambulance trip to the hospital

July 1951: One Saturday I went to Mollie's home for some much needed relaxation with family and friends. As I went to bed that night, I did not feel well. When I woke up the next morning I was sick as a dog, had a terrific backache, headache, stiff neck, sore throat, and high fever. All day I tossed and moaned with pain. At that time the polio epidemic was in full swing, but I never thought it was in my range of possibilities.

Mollie's family was so worried about me. By 4 p.m. my fever had risen to 104, so mother decided to call Dr. G. and ask him to make a house-call since I felt too sick to go to his office. An hour later, after he examined me, he took precautions against me having polio – he called the ambulance and had them take me to the student infirmary at the hospital. That was a new experience for me. With the siren howling, the driver raced through town and arrived at the hospital about 6 p.m.

Later I wrote in my journal: *I joined four other nursing students who were also patients there in the infirmary. Marty and Patty both had appendectomies. Ardis had a bad stomachache; turned out she needed to have her appendix out, too. Jane had a tonsillectomy. What camaraderie for all of us to be sick together.*

Sunday morning I was feeling pretty rough, temp 102.4, and still aching all over. After more medicine to reduce the pain and fever, I felt more comfortable. Mollie's family came to visit and cheer me up in the afternoon. How kind they have been to me! I have been very blessed.

Mrs. K. came to the infirmary to visit us, and we all felt like fools. In her teasing way she suggested we were all just pretending to be sick to get out of work. It was hard to tell if she was teasing or serious.

Dr. H. joked with me by asking if I had stuck the thermometer against the radiator yesterday. Wednesday he allowed me to get out of bed for the first time and walk in the hall. Thursday morning he discharged me. Friday it seemed strange to be back at work again after a whole week with who knows what. What do you suppose was wrong with me? I wasn't given a clear diagnosis, but probably the flu bug hit me hard and laid me low. I'm just so thankful I didn't have polio.

It proved to be very interesting to be a patient and have to follow doctors' and nurses' orders. That's one way I can learn to empathize with my patients and be more understanding.

Moving again

In mid-August, Mrs. K. informed those of us junior students who lived in Forney House that we had to move to a different dorm to make room for the new students that were scheduled to come in a few weeks. Oh dear! Did I really have to move again – this would be the fourth time in a year.

I was scheduled to move half a block down the street to the Bowan House nurses' residence. I just couldn't force myself to pack up my stuff. I didn't want to leave dear Ruthie, my roommate for the last six months. But it had to happen. Orders come down from on high. As I sorted my stuff, I was appalled at how much junk I had collected in the short time I lived there.

More Men's Medical evening duty

July 28, 1951: *Oh diary, I'm nearer to crying than I have been for a long time! Maybe it's PMS? I was looking forward to seeing Carl on my day off. He called a short time ago and said it didn't suit for him to come this weekend because he has to give a presentation at church.*

Again, it's one of those times when I'm tempted to quit this program altogether. Such crazy hours to work and so many lost leisure hours. Now I really do feel like blubbering – so I think I will do just that.

The next afternoon, I felt a little better when I went on duty. It helped to cry it out the evening before. Even though I still felt despondent, I was able to care for the patients as usual. The bantering and camaraderie that went on between patients and staff uplifted my spirits.

Dear little 90-year-old Abner was so cute. When he cracked his jokes with a straight face, we had to laugh and it cheered everybody up for a while.

July 30, 1951 Evening shift: *After 7 o'clock, Marla and I were trying to settle everybody down when everything decided to happen at once. Mr. Gibson was restless, so we put bedrails on for him so he wouldn't fall out of bed. About 9:30, he crawled out over the end of the bed and voided all over the floor. What a messy puddle that was to clean up. It's a miracle he didn't fall and break a hip!*

Pappy, a.k.a. "Santa Claus," with his long white beard, decided to crawl out over the end of his bed and walk all the way to the bathroom at the end of the ward when he was supposed to be on complete bedrest.

Mr. Spader was quite a pill, too; he wouldn't keep his oxygen mask on so we practically had to "special" him so he could breathe.

All this was in addition to our usual duties, admissions, and discharges. When we left at 11:30 p.m., I was so dead tired I didn't know if I could even drag myself up the steps to my room.

The next evening: *10:30 p.m. I'll start writing this in the nurses' station on Men's Medical with all our patients settled in their beds for the night, hopefully. My dear friend Gracie and I work fast together. Right now, for a change, everything is calm and peaceful in the ward. None of the men are critically ill right now. Some of them are more congenial than others. So far we've had a moderately busy shift tonight – five discharges and three admissions.*

Last night Mr. Jones had what he described as "terrible pain", so I gave him a placebo (a sugar pill) that the doctor had ordered for him.

This morning the nurse reported that he slept all night. It's so interesting to see how placebos can work psychologically.

A young fellow, 19 years old, attempted suicide by ingesting rat poison because his girlfriend ditched him. We gave him something to make him vomit and also some yukky stuff to counteract that poison. He's quite sick, but his vital signs are improving and he's vomiting less frequently so I think he will survive. This was his second attempt. If he does try it again, he'll probably succeed. Third time is the charm, they say. I hope he gets some help to deal with his emotional pain.

Admitting emergencies

After getting off work so late the night before, I didn't feel like putting forth that much effort the next morning. I decided to conserve my energy for duty the next evening, so I slept late and just puttered around till it was time to go to work at 3 p.m.

I was glad to be well rested when I went back on duty the next afternoon because the whole ward was in an uproar. Gloria reported to us that the night nurse had a really rough night. She admitted three accident cases.

August 4, 1951: *The first admission was a young fellow who fell asleep while driving and ran the car off the road. He suffered a shattered leg and severe internal injuries. We had to prep him for a stat (immediate) surgery. His wife was with him and was badly injured. She was admitted to Women's Surgical and died about 15 minutes after admission. Poor guy, he was devastated when they told him she had died.*

The second admission was a fellow who fell down while he was dead drunk and hit his head on a rock. He was admitted unconscious. X-rays showed he had a skull fracture and internal bleeding. We sent him to surgery, also.

The third accident happened when the young intoxicated driver was driving the wrong way on a one-way street and hit another car head-on. X-rays showed he suffered a fractured pelvis, and all we could do for him that night was keep him comfortable with pain medicine. It was a miracle all of them weren't killed. I never heard how those in the other car fared.

Relaxing off duty

Three of us nurses in Bowan House were on evening duty at the same time. We stirred up the most hilarious antics in our dorm after we were off duty at 11:30 p.m. It was pitiful how silly and giggly we could act after needing to be so professional and proper for eight hours. Somehow we had to let out the tension and frustration. We tried to keep from waking up our fellow nurses who had to get up for early duty the next morning. If they were still awake, they were probably irritated with us. Sometimes they joined us in our silliness.

August 5, 1951: *Talk about wasting time. I never did so much lazing around and goofing off in all my life as I have this week on evening duty. Today, mind you, I stayed in bed all morning listening to a church service and good music on the radio until time to go to work at 2:45 p.m. That is awful on a Sunday. Should I feel guilty? Of course, I should. But I don't. I was glad I had extra rest before going back to work on the hectic ward.*

One thing I liked about being on evening duty – I could get up when I pleased and putter around till time to go to work at 3 p.m. Another plus about evening duty – only one graduate worked with two of us students. The pace on evening duty was usually less hectic except when we admitted or discharged patients.

On the day shift, there were usually too many people roaming around: doctors, supervisors, students, interns, orderlies, housekeeping people. We almost tripped over each other. Some were harder to get along with than others and they often scolded us students for what seemed like petty incidents. Surely the heat and humidity made staff and patients more irritable, too. The summer weather was so hot in the middle of the day – just like a sauna in the hospital. The perspiration just poured off of us as we worked.

Some good news – my best friend Mollie was accepted into the nursing program here. She and I had a long visit the day she came to be measured for her student uniforms. We were so glad for a chance to be together again.

Loving long-awaited vacation

My two weeks of vacation began the second week of August and I could sleep to my heart's content, spend quality time with my adopted family, and have fun times with my friends. Oh, it was like heaven.

One morning while the rest of the family was off doing other things, I was by myself enjoying a late breakfast in the kitchen. The milkman came to the door to deliver the day's supply of milk and later the bakery person drove up in his delivery wagon to see what bread, rolls, or pies I might want to buy. I felt like I was the lady of the house, but I didn't have money to buy anything.

In that area of rural Pennsylvania, fresh meat, vegetables, fruits, bread, milk, ice cream, etc. were peddled and delivered house to house in open-sided trucks or wagons. It was a very unique and handy service.

Mid-afternoon, Carl picked me up and took me to his home a few miles away. There I helped him clean eggs while we chatted and caught up with each other's life. His folks raised a lot of chickens and took the eggs to market every week. Later his Aunt Elma and Uncle Charles invited us over for one of her scrumptious fish suppers.

Where I grew up in Kansas we never ate fish except maybe an occasional can of tuna or salmon. During the three years in Pennsylvania I ate fresh fish more times than I could count. That's because we lived so close to the ocean.

August 8, 1951: *Today I went with the family to the first session of the annual church camp meeting. Honestly, such carryings-on as they have there. I never saw the likes of it before. It was an extreme version of what people did during revival meetings in my home church where I grew up. During the service, several people got "blessed" at the same time. They screamed at the top of their voices, tearfully raced up and* *down the aisles, waved white lacy handkerchiefs, and danced around like mad people. Some even spoke in an unintelligible language. I wondered if they do this for attention or to prove their devotion? I don't understand this kind of radical emotionalism. I guess some people need to express themselves this way, but my emotions aren't like that. The quiet, peaceful communion with God out in nature is more meaningful to me. It just shows that we are all different but can love God in different ways. Something to ponder.*

August 19, 1951: *Carl asked me to go along to help teach a childrens' Sunday school class at the little mountain church where he had held vacation Bible school and church services in early summer. The dear children were so eager to learn the Bible verses, sing the choruses, and listen with rapt attention to the Bible stories we told.*

He and I had other quality times together during my vacation but, as always, we had to say goodbye. Sigh. Such is life full of let-downs and partings. Having such good fellowship together, I allowed myself to get so buried in loving him that each goodbye was painful. I wondered if he had that trouble, too; I wanted to ask him sometime when we were together. The time came all too soon when my vacation was over and I came back to work and study again.

Chapter 13
The Diet Kitchen

Working in dietary department

August 22, 1951: *After vacation, my next assignment was four weeks in the Diet Kitchen. Monday morning I woke up to the abrasive jangle of my trusty alarm clock at 6 a.m. It brought me back to reality very fast. I quickly bathed and donned my clean, stiffly starched, scratchy uniform for the first time in two weeks. It seemed so strange to wear it again after enjoying casual summer clothes.*

Before I went to breakfast at 6:45, I ran over to check my work schedule that day. Just as I suspected, I wasn't scheduled to be at the diet kitchen until 10 a.m. so I high-tailed it back to my room and crawled in my almost-still-warm bed to catch a few more winks. I pulled the covers over my head hoping to shut out the loud, irritating, construction noises.

Constant grinding and hammering sounds are due to a major construction project. When finished, it will almost double the bed capacity of the hospital. Even with all the noise, I snoozed for almost two hours. That extra shut-eye felt so good. I was ready to face whatever was ahead.

Nutrition class flop

After one of the nutrition classes, I wrote: *Mrs. M. seemed to be a very amiable teacher. Cindy and I were partners in the nutrition lab learning to prepare simple breakfast trays for patients. Our first assignment was to squeeze oranges for juice, make tea and toast, then judge each other's patient tray for neatness.*

You should have seen the terrible flop of cupcakes we made the next week in class. We had to use spoons to eat them out of the muffin tins because they were so crumbly. It was ridiculously funny. Even our instructor laughed with us. None of us could figure out why they flopped. Maybe the recipe was wrong or the oven wasn't set right.

Maybe we didn't get the ingredients measured right. Or they flopped because we were all so keyed up over the tough anatomy & physiology final exam we took later in the day.

I was so relieved after that terrible exam I was tempted to scream at the top of my lungs all the way down Broadway Ave. If we have many more like that, I'll go batty for sure. I'd better start studying, though, for the next final in microbiology coming up. If that's on a Monday and I have to cram during my precious weekend off, I'm going to do something drastic. Can't imagine what that would be. A person has to be so serious around here.

In the four weeks working in Diet Kitchen, my buddies and I learned how to plan and prepare various types of diets for patients with different needs. The first week we made special diets: low salt, soft, fat-free, diabetic, pureed, clear liquids, and full liquids. That was a complicated job, but we got through it.

The second week, I was assigned to do the cooking for the special diets. I feared something terrible would happen – the cereal would be lumpy, eggs hard boiled, potatoes would scorch or boil over. Since I didn't hear of any deaths during that time, my cooking must have agreed with them. I made quite a few dumb mistakes, though, but that was the only way I knew how to learn something new. Our instructor was patient with us novices. One or two times she was crabby and out of sorts, but that was to be expected. My other student buddies didn't know how to cook any better than I did. It was a pleasant experience overall. We learned to go with the flow, and we laughed a lot.

On my way to pick up some diet trays on Men's Medical ward, my friend Josie flagged me down and informed me that a box of chocolates was left there in the nurses' station with my name on it! Who could they possibly be from, I wondered? What a surprise when I opened the box – they were from Mr. Waters, the patient who said he'd give my boyfriend a discount on gasoline from his service station. My, oh my, those chocolates were much too close to resist temptation. I shared them with my buddies on dorm that evening. Such sweet delicacies they were!

September 9, 1951: *Such a frustrating day as this has been. I hope there will never be another one like it. I cooked dinner in the Diet Kitchen today and it ended in such a disaster. It turned out that I made too much rice pudding and not enough apple cobbler. I was so glad when it was over.*

In spite of it all, four weeks in Diet Kitchen went by fast. I was definitely ready for a change of scenery. It wasn't exactly my cup of tea.

Back to the books

More journaling: *Mrs. K. was in an unusually good mood in our professional problems class yesterday. Her moods are so changeable and unpredictable! Much of the time she's grouchy, has a frown on her face, and chews us out about every little thing. I usually dreaded meeting her anywhere, never knowing what mood she would be in.*

This time she actually kept us laughing. We were super happy when she told us we could all have an extra midnight curfew this Friday night. Maybe she got a raise in pay, or something equally exciting, that caused her to be so cheerful and generous.

I'm exhausted now, ready for a good night's sleep, hopefully. I plan to spend the weekend at Mollie's home. Carl and I may have a chance to be together again after these many weeks. He's so very busy with his studies at college. Even if I don't see him it will be good just to get away from this stuffy hospital. We bury ourselves here week in and week out and need a change of scenery frequently.

September 12, 1951: *Hot, humid summer days have flown by, and September is upon us already. We are hit with classes and tough tests again. Another big word surfaced in OB-GYN class one day: "pseudomucuscystoadenocarcinomatous." Hey, that's 33 letters. I'm not exaggerating either. We even had it on the big test. It refers to cancerous, mucus-laden cysts on the ovaries that imitate other types of cancer. I had no idea the medical field was so full of big words. There were many more long ones that demanded our memory banks to work* *on over-time. Those two years of Latin classes in high school are also helping me better understand the medical terminology.*

As often as three days a week, I was scheduled for a split shift. That meant I worked from 7 a.m. until noon. After lunch I usually went to my room and took a nap before going back to work from 3:30 until 7 p.m. No one was fond of split shifts mainly because it didn't allow us to attend evening activities – just another one of those things that was expected of us and it was out of our control.

I soon got into a very bad habit of sleeping during those three hours off duty. All I wanted to do by that time was flop down on my bed that looked oh so tempting. In my head, I knew I should be doing other things, but when my lower back and legs ached so fiercely I needed to relax.

Part Three

Becoming Intermediate Nurses

Chapter 14
Taking Another Big Step:
The First Black Band for our Caps

Joy of joys, a small miracle took place in morning chapel on Monday, September 10, 1951. At the end of this one year anniversary of our entrance into these hallowed halls of learning, our class celebrated this long anticipated stepping stone to success – our junior year ended and we entered the ecstatic status of intermediate student nurses for the next twelve months.

To mark this passage, Mrs. K. gave each of us one jet black, velvet ribbon one quarter inch wide and about ten inches long to fasten on to our starched caps. That black ribbon signaled to everyone we met that we had actually progressed to the intermediate status. Hallelujah.

It was sobering, though, because it also meant that now we were expected to be more qualified to take on more responsibility. We could now demonstrate all the knowledge and skill the faculty had poured into us during the past year. One year down and two more to go. Yep, we were making progress ever so slowly.

What a hilarious feeling to know that next year at this time we would become seniors. A year after that we would take the final leap to graduation, state board exams and become registered nurses.

This was also an exciting day for others – the seniors were finished with their three-year program and the new probies were beginning their three year journey. This included my soul-sister Mollie who decided to enter the nursing program here. Mrs. K. gave them a big lecture on respecting the older students. That included us. It gave our class a strange but exhilarating sensation when they held the doors open for us and decorously allowed us to walk ahead of them in the cafeteria line. Such were their orders from the Madam.

The probies enviously looked up to us in our uniforms and wished they were as far along as we were. That was exactly what we did last year with the intermediate and senior students. Had it really been a whole year since we were the lowly probationers around here and needed lots of encouragement?

Mollie, bless her heart, had always been gung ho to take on new experiences. This time though she came to my room to lament how lost and overwhelmed she was feeling with this one. This was a new kind of challenge. Her chin quivered and her eyes welled up with big tears. I offered her a tissue to dry those tears at the same time I offered what I hoped were comforting words to her. I assured her that I'd be her sounding board:

"You can cry on my shoulder anytime. I keep crying towels handy. You will feel depressed and anxious from time to time just like I have many times this past year. Don't wallow in it, though. Find someone to talk to."

This was what Gracie had said to me when I felt so discouraged at first.

The next week again she was feeling in a blue mood after being introduced to the beginning classes.

"Oh I just don't think I can do this," she moaned.

I gave her another one of my pep talks, encouraging her to hang in there even though the adjustment was so hard. In an attempt to ease her anxiety I told her, "You will gradually get used to how the professors throw a lot at you all at once."

(She successfully completed the three year nursing program and had a rewarding career for many years.)

Taking advantage of schedule change

September 23, 1951: *Miracles have been happening to me lately. I really wanted to go to hear Carl's music group give a concert at 2 p.m. today, but I was scheduled to work a split shift. I politely asked the nurse supervisor, Miss B., if I could be off from 1-4 instead of 12-3:30.*

*At first she said, "No, I don't have enough staff to do that."
I didn't want to be demanding since I had asked for a special favor
yesterday. I said, "O.K., I just thought I would ask."*

*I was prepared to tell him I couldn't be there but at 10 o'clock Miss S.,
one of the 3-11 nurses, called in sick. That meant Miss B. could shuffle
staff around, send one of us off duty at 11 a.m., come back at 7 p.m.
and work until 11 p.m. I silently prayed that she would choose me, that
way I would have plenty of time to go to the concert and be back in
time to finish off the evening shift. Sure enough, a few minutes later
Miss B. took me aside and said I could be off from 11a.m.-7 p.m. So
now I had the whole afternoon off. I was overjoyed. I called to tell
Carl, and he too was glad that I wouldn't have to rush back right after
their program.*

Chapter 15
Night Duty on Men's Surgical Ward

Five weeks on Men's Surgical Ward – one week on day duty and four weeks on night duty – was my next clinical assignment. Working with the patients provided lots of grist for my (almost) daily journal.

September 19, 1951: *Elderly Mr. Conn is quite the character. He is forever trying to climb over the bedrails. When I look down the center of the ward and see his hospital gown flapping around his bare bottom and his skinny bare legs flying around in midair, it looks ridiculously funny. So far, we've been able to catch him before he falls and injures himself.*

Mr. Steh can be a problem, too. He hollers for a blanket or demands a urinal every few minutes. The other patients are younger, cheerful, and easy to care for.

My back aches a lot tonight – I must have strained it today lifting those old men around! They are both lead weights.

September 20, 1951: *Today Mr. Conn was ambitiously trying to crawl over the rails again, so we tried shackling his feet to the bed with strips of sheeting. That little old man is so strong, and he tore them right off.*

He complained loudly, "You ____'s [expletive] are taking my freedom away and I'm going to get the law after you!"

I said to Gracie who was working with me, "Just let him try to sue us."

Starting night duty

Here was my chance to have a fling at night duty to see what it was like. It would either make me or break me. I didn't know if I would make it through the nights without getting sleepy.

September 22, 1951: *Only two more mornings that I have to get up for work before I go on night shift. I'm a bit anxious and hope I can do it o.k. I'm looking forward to something different than anything I've done before.*

Just before going to work I lamented in my journal about my futile attempts to sleep during the day.

September 24, 1951: *I was so disgusted at myself today. I tried to sleep but no sleep would come. I think I was too excited about going on night duty tonight for the first time. When it was time to go to work at 11 p.m., I was already tired. What a bummer. Wish me luck.*

It was so different to work all through the night. The ward was pretty busy because a fresh appendectomy came from the O.R. at about 1 a.m. Monitoring him helped keep me awake.

Soon after midnight, we admitted a critically ill, suicidal patient. He had ingested Phenobarbital and exposed himself to carbon monoxide poisoning. It was nip and tuck there for a while. We feared that he would not make it out alive. I assessed him to be mentally confused, too. He made it through the night. I was so thankful he didn't die on my shift.

Men's Surgical was a hard place to work with a lot of critically ill surgical patients. I felt totally inadequate and nervous in situations like that. I was glad to have Miss R., a new graduate, as my charge nurse. I was more at ease with her because I had known her when she was a student.

The following days were so chopped up with classes that it was hard to get enough sleep during the day. Besides that, the construction project on the new part of the hospital was so noisy. Bang bang, buzz buzz. Mary offered me her bed to sleep in while she was on day duty, so that's what I did. What a generous offer that was. Her room was the farthest from the construction noises. I can't say it helped all that much, though. The loud noises still bothered me, but I soon learned to tune them out a bit.

Miss G., the night supervisor, was fairly easy to get along with. Bob was the night orderly. He was a nice chap who came around to give the pre-surgical enemas to the men in the early mornings.

The next night I felt miserable when it was time to go on duty having had only three hours sleep that day. I had tried to sleep after class but I was too tense and couldn't relax. Could I stay awake for the next eight hours, or would I walk around like a zombie?

I wondered what excitement was in store for us the next night. Would Pappy Conn stay in bed for me? Or would he hobble to the bathroom several times, fall, and break a hip? Mr. Steh was a nuisance, too, waking the other patients with his constant yelling.

September 28, 1951: *I hardly know where to begin to tell about last night's excitement. While we were eating supper we heard about this fellow who had been blasting a rock. The story as we heard it was that he got too close to the dynamite and it went off in his face and upper body. I was pretty sure he would be admitted later on Men's Surgical. Doctors worked on him a long time in the O.R.*

Sure enough, about 1 a.m. the O.R. staff brought him to our ward. What a terrible sight he was. The only visible portion of his bandaged face was the end of his nose. His left hand was amputated, his left leg had a huge hole in it, his left eye had been removed, and his lips were sutured shut. He had I.V. fluid going in one arm and a blood transfusion going in his other arm. Never have I seen such a mangled human being.

I was working all alone this time caring for the eighteen other sick patients. Quickly I called Miss G., the night supervisor, to ask for help. She sent another nurse to help me. About 4 a.m. he quit breathing, so I called for the emergency crash cart team. They rushed around like mad, hoping to resuscitate him but to no avail. At 4:45 a.m. he was pronounced dead – a sudden death, to be sure – but at least he was spared a long and painful recovery as well as a badly scarred face and torso. I felt very sad for his family as they grieved the loss of their loved one.

As I made my hourly rounds of the other patients with my flashlight, I discovered old Mr. Herzt was incontinent and lying in a wet bed. I cleaned him up and changed his linens. Then Mr. Geig, who had attempted suicide, had a petit mal seizure. The doctor on call came rushing in and together we got him under control with medication. In tense situations like these I hardly knew which way to turn, but it sure kept me awake. I was totally exhausted when I went off duty.

I had just barely said my prayers, crawled into my comfy bed, and was nearly asleep when Miss Kensy, the day shift supervisor, called to tell me that I neglected to complete a couple of charts. Oh my, was I ever jarred and upset at myself. Reluctantly I got up, impatiently threw on my uniform again and went back to finish those d---d charts! As the saying goes, "No rest for the weary."

October 1, 1951: *Last night was a hectic night. Mr. M. gave up the fight for life about 1 a.m. We didn't expect him to die just yet. That gave me a very chilly feeling. Mr. Steh has gone home, and that's a relief off my hands. I got so provoked at him sometimes with his constant yelling and restlessness.*

I got some sleep today for a change in spite of the construction noises. Jan and I went to bed at 11 am and didn't get up till about 9:30 pm – just a little while ago. Now I'm feeling up to another night of – who knows what?

October 9, 1951: *Night duty is too much nervous tension for me. Friday morning I just went to Gracie's room and bawled like a baby. The critical patients have me on edge because I never know when they will die. Miss G. is so persnickety, too, which gets me all in a dither. Weekend nights were often quieter compared to some of the others.*

Surviving night shift

October 25, 1951: *Can you forgive me for not writing in you for almost 3 weeks? Studies have taken up so much of my time, and I've been very negligent in writing lately. Plus, I have to grab sleep whenever I can.*

It happened again – one morning after going off duty, I was already fast asleep in my comfy bed when the day shift supervisor called to tell me I needed to come back and finish my work. In my sleepy state I couldn't fathom what I had not done. Come to find out, in all my busyness I had neglected to empty a patient's bedpan before I went off duty. She said the day shift nurse found it in the patient's private room on a chair with the usual canvas bedpan cover over it. Of course, she scolded me thoroughly for this lapse in my performance and ordered me to come back and empty it. Humiliated, I dutifully got up, dressed and went back to finish what needed to be done. I didn't get much sleep that day because classes took up most of the afternoon. Such is life as a student nurse.

It was unusual that an intermediate student would be scheduled alone on night duty. Usually a graduate worked along with a student. Not enough graduates stayed around, I guess. I had to call on the night supervisor quite often if there was a crisis.

Juggling both night duty (a full 48 hour week) and classes too proved to be more difficult than I expected. Studies took up more and more of my time, so sleep time was sacrificed. Two of the classes – gynecology and obstetrics – were heavy but extremely interesting. They furnished many juicy tidbits of conversation for our off-duty gab sessions.

Night shift messed up my sleep pattern big time when classes started again in September. Sleep deprivation combined with heavy-duty study and classes made it so nerve-wracking for me. That may be why my efficiency report was disappointing. Miss G. graded me low on the few mistakes I made and didn't consider my improvements. Not everything depended on her opinion, but it did challenge me to keep improving my nursing skills. After four weeks I was very glad to get off night duty. Thank God I made it through. It was an intense learning experience, to say the least.

Chapter 16
Women's Medical Ward

Grappling with seven weeks of hard work

I was stunned when I found out my next assignment was Women's Medical Ward for seven weeks of day-evening-night shifts! That was a hard place to work, too. We had some real nice patients most of the time. For instance, the first day I worked there Mrs. Hale slipped a $1 bill in my hand to pay for my bus fare home. That was a real help since I was low on funds.

October 31, 1951: *This has been one very tiring day shift on Women's Medical. Today it wasn't only the work that got on my nerves it was the staff people. Miss Brown, the charge nurse, wasn't too bad, but Ms. Lese just irked my liver. I was working as fast as I could when she scolded me for not changing Nancy's bed linens before I went to class. Then I realized I had missed seeing Nancy's name on my assignment sheet. Oh dear! After I changed her bedding, I hustled off to class but it made me late. Seems like I can't win for losing sometimes. Why do I end up doing such dumb things?*

Later, I was merely getting a drink of water from the kitchenette when Miss Band walked in. She looked at me rather quizzically and said scornfully, "Hmm, Are you loafing again, Miss Minter? I hear you are pretty good at it."

A feather could have knocked me over just then. I was so humiliated. As I tried to collect my wits about me, I seethed with anger inside. Grrr! You can't even blink an eye around this place before someone jumps down your throat about some little thing. Truthfully, I'm getting sick of it. It wouldn't take much for me to quit now and forever. (Oh, I forgot my vow to not complain or threaten to quit. OK, I take that back.)

November 1, 1951: *Oh diary, this was my only day off this week and, wouldn't you know, we had three classes so I had to stay here at the hospital all day! Life can be so unfair. I've got to start finding some* *joy around this place or I'll go bonkers. Maybe I'm there already and just don't know it.*

We're having a Halloween party later tonight, so I'll see if maybe the ghosts and goblins can boost my spirits and help me feel better.

Almost half the patients on Women's Medical had psychiatric problems. Dr. Buri, the psychiatrist, made his rounds every morning. Two attempted suicides from barbiturate poisonings were in beds right beside each other. I wondered if they compared notes. Another lady was a hypochondriac convinced she was terribly sick. All kinds of tests showed nothing was wrong with her.

Two new admissions were brought in which made the ward nearly full again. That evening we weren't as busy since several of our difficult patients had been discharged. It wouldn't be long, though, till others were admitted to take their place.

November 10, 1951: *Dear journal, remember I said the quiet ward couldn't last very long? Well, tonight was worse than we could ever have anticipated. Two patients were admitted by ambulance at the same time about 9:45 p.m. One woman was a profuse vaginal bleeder who had to be prepped for surgery.*

The other woman had a CVA (stroke) and was very close to death. What a terrible commotion. We couldn't get oxygen equipment set up fast enough for this lady and she almost died on us. Because she was so very obese, we couldn't roll her over to undress her and put a hospital gown on her. We ended up having to cut her clothes off of her. Her poor husband was almost hysterical. He frantically fussed at us to work faster until we were at our wits' end. In spite of our best efforts, we found out the next morning that she died during the night.

The ambulance brought another attempted suicide patient – Mrs. Mavoy. She was such a tough looking character, terribly sick, vomited yukky black stuff, and had a horrible body odor that almost made me sick to my stomach. She had swallowed an unknown quantity of mercuric chloride tablets. The policeman told us her husband had smuggled the tablets to her while she was a prisoner at the jail. I spent time with her while IV fluids were infusing in her veins. She asked me questions about soul salvation and heaven, so I talked to her about God's love. She asked if I would pray with her, so that's what I did. When I went to work the next day, I discovered she died early that morning! I was glad I had that one and only opportunity to speak to her.

Playing tricks on the doctor

One evening, Dr. Grant, the medical resident, was making his usual rounds. He had the habit of leaving his smoldering pipe on our charting table, and it would stink up the small space. This time Fran and I decided to play a trick on him. She used a paper towel to gingerly pick up the smelly thing and lock it in the narcotic box.

When he came back to look for it he became very frustrated. He couldn't remember where he had put it, and he had a hard time getting along without it. We confessed that we had hidden it, but refused to give it back to him until after we gave report to the night nurse and were ready to go off duty. He took our teasing very well, though. At least he learned his lesson – do not leave your pipe lying around these nurses.

Uproar on the ward

November 17, 1951, 11:30 p.m.: *I found the ward in an uproar when I went on duty at 3 p.m. Several patients were being discharged at the same time, and an out-of-town ambulance arrived with a patient who was suffering grand mal seizures. She had bitten her tongue badly during a seizure and was spitting out blood. I quickly prepared the medication the doctor ordered to decrease the seizures.*

By 7 p.m. everything was pretty well under control. About 8 p.m. we admitted an elderly patient with acute upper abdominal pain who needed an admission bath and a lot of extra care. The poor lady is as deaf as a doorknob and terribly frightened because she couldn't understand us and we couldn't communicate with her about what we were going to do for her. We ended up writing notes and that helped her to be less agitated.

About 8:30 p.m., Drs. Mosse and Appello decided they needed to remove Ms. Mell's gallbladder so we flew madly around to prep her for surgery. As I finished my charting and was ready to give report to the night nurse, the O.R. staff brought her back to the ward right at 11 p.m. in critical condition with oxygen, blood, and glucose running. You can imagine how fast I had to dash around. Miss G., the night supervisor, called for an extra nurse to come in to monitor the critical surgery patient. That was a great help.

I gave report to the night nurse, and it was almost midnight when I finally dragged myself wearily over to the nurses' residence. I didn't know if I could make it to my room. Slowly I climbed up five steps to the porch and ten more steps to my room on second floor. I was so tired I could hardly wait to yank my uniform off, jump into my jammies, and flop down on my comfy bed.

As I was undressing, I discovered the keys to the narcotic box were still in my uniform pocket. I had forgotten to give them to the night nurse! Thankfully I wasn't in bed yet this time. I put that scratchy, sweaty uniform back on and literally ran over to the ward to give them to her. By then my head was in total spin mode. I kept wondering, "Why do I do such dumb stuff?" There seems to be no credible answer except maybe fatigue from overwork.

Right now, my brain feels like it is sloshing around like a whirlpool in my cranial cavity. I hope I can turn it off and go to sleep. I'm not often this dead tired. Maybe it's because I feel a terrible head cold coming on. I think I'll stay home from church in the morning. Sleep will do more good for me than church this time.

November 18, 1951, 11:30 p.m.: *I felt like a wrung-out dishrag all day today, so guess what – I stayed in bed and doctored my cold. Twinges of guilt coursed through my brain when I decided to stay home from church today. I was able to study a couple of hours for two upcoming exams.*

When I went on duty at 3 p.m., I was feeling a little bit better. I was so glad this shift would be the end of my evening duty spree. I definitely prefer the 7-3 day duty or 11-7 night duty hours because then I can go to more evening social activities. But the powers that be never give us the choice. Whether we want to or not, our superiors expect us to work the whole range of shifts: days-evenings-nights give us maximum experience.

Ms. Mell died this afternoon. We knew she was a poor operative risk, but she died sooner than we expected.

Ms. Gaum did a very unique thing – she pulled out her Foley catheter, balloon and all. That must have been painful. I had to reinsert another catheter. She yelled and screamed briefly until I gave her a backrub. It didn't take her long to quiet down and fall asleep. I used soft restraints to tie her hands to the bedrail so she wouldn't pull it out again.

(Restraining a patient is not legal any more. Some hospitals use a monitor to signal when a patient is becoming agitated or in danger of falling. If they pull out their tube/s, then we just put them back in again.)

Monday I went back to day duty and two dreaded tests, gynecology and orthopedics. I studied hard for those dumb tests. They turned out to be fairly easy.

The next weekend it was great to have a Saturday off with NO classes. Finally I could relax and sleep in till 9:30 and be home ALL day. At my dental appointment the dentist found three rather small cavities. He said it would cost almost $20 to fix them satisfactorily. Then I had to figure out how to pay for it. Voilá! It was my lucky day to be offered a babysitting job.

November 21, 1951: *On duty at 7 a.m., off 12-3:30 – a split shift. Naomi and I went downtown to get drapes and a lampshade for our newly decorated room during our break.*

In pediatrics class from 9-11 with Dr. H., we studied the most effective principles of discipline with problem children. It was an engrossing child psychology course.

When I went back to work at 3:30 p.m., the place was so busy we didn't get off duty till 7:30 p.m. Most of my time was spent monitoring one critical patient – Mrs. Forry. We did all we could to reduce her fever but without success. She died of a severe case of pneumonia about 6 p.m. with a temp of 107.4.

One Saturday I filled in on an evening shift for someone who had called in sick. I was glad to have an excuse not to go to the Saturday night dance with the other girls. That was the underlying reason I felt out of sorts all evening. (Many times I wanted to learn to dance, but dancing was forbidden as I was growing up.)

Once again my feelings spilled over in my journal: *Ms. R. was certainly a pill tonight. She thinks she is the only patient we have to take care of, and she reported us to her doctor because we don't cater to her every whim.*

Before long, her doctor called the nurses' station and said in his croaky voice, "Why aren't you taking better care of my patient?"

I had a strong urge to bark right back at him, "Dr. P., you can come up here and babysit your demanding patient any time."

Thankfully, I controlled my naughty impulses and didn't act on my true feelings. That would have meant disaster for me as a student. So I went to her, took time to listen to her concerns, gave her a calming backrub, and made sure she was comfortable. Before long she was sound asleep.

I was furious, too, at Kevin, the orderly on call. At 4 o'clock I called him and politely asked him to come to catheterize a male patient who was in extreme pain in one of the private rooms. He retorted sarcastically that he was scheduled to go off duty at 5 p.m. and had a date with his girlfriend. If he did that catheterization, it means he would have to work overtime.

I pleaded with him, emphasizing how urgent it was to relieve the patient of his discomfort. He continued to refuse until I said as calmly as I could even though I was seething inside, "Then I will have to call the doctor."

He realized that I was serious and would do just that. Grudgingly he relented and reluctantly came to catheterize the poor fellow. His pouty attitude permeated the whole ward as he grumbled about these bossy nurses.

I could have grouched right back at him about egotistical orderlies who think they are so superior and entitled to their own wishes over the needs of the patients. Honestly, in my opinion, he is too conceited to be an asset to this institution.

November 29, 1951: *Today was a pretty good shift on Women's Medical. Ms. Hartman was admitted, and at first glance we thought she had a stroke. When the doctor examined her more carefully, he diagnosed her mentally deranged and in the catatonic stage of dementia.*

Dr. O'Donnell did a sternal puncture on another lady, and I was designated to take the tissue sample to the lab to test for a blood dyscrasia (abnormality). Each of these patients had conditions that I had not seen up close before now. It was a very interesting shift.

We admitted another poor soul who tried to commit suicide by barbiturates. What is it with all these suicides lately? Must be something in the water. Probably just the sad state of our world – people don't have any hope for the future if they don't know God's love.

We had a horrible final in dermatology. I'm sure I flunked it. If the truth be known, I really don't care much. Let them take away my one precious overnight privilege in a month. We don't get days off anyway when we have to stay at the hospital for so many classes.

Our spirits were lifted a bit when we discovered that Mr. Hooten brought the nurses a huge can of Minder's potato chips and Mrs. Sanford sent us a big box of See's candy – the best. So we will all get pleasingly plump over those goodies.

December 1, 1951: *Our dermatology test came back. I barely passed the thing. Personally, I don't give a hoot what grade I got just so I passed. We were all relieved to have that difficult subject behind us. Now I'm totally exhausted.*

Chapter 17
Beginning Maternity, Nursery, Labor and Delivery Rotation

With great anticipation I looked forward to a four month assignment on the Maternity Unit. It turned out to be a whole new adventure. I knew delivering babies and caring for new mothers and newborns would be a lot different from medical/surgical nursing. There was a downside, though. The majority of the time students were scheduled for evening and night duty. That fact in itself was hard to accept.

During this assignment, I was scheduled to work two weeks of day duty in labor and delivery, two weeks of day duty with babies in the nurseries and with the mothers on the post-partum floors, six weeks of evening duty (3 p.m. - 11 p.m.) and six weeks of night duty (11 p.m. - 7 a.m.) all divided between labor and delivery rooms, three nurseries, and three floors of post-partum patients.

The maternity wing was built in 1929 and added 80 more beds to the hospital – 54 for maternity patients and 26 for ward patients. In l953 the hospital recorded a record of 3,141 births (LGH: 100 years of caring p.61).

Nursery Duty

January 4, 1952, My first impressions: *Maternity and infant nurseries are wonderful – so far. At first I was nervous about how I would handle a tiny baby. It's been nearly 9 years since my youngest brother was born. My anxieties were alleviated somewhat when Mrs. Nance, the nurse who oriented me, said babies aren't as breakable as they look. It was a matter of learning safe ways to handle them.*

There's so much to learn. My goodness, I can hardly keep everything under one hat. She did a great job of teaching me, so I think I will catch on quickly. I just have to learn by doing and by being reminded of little details. Just now we have 20 newborns in 2nd floor nursery. When I went to work this morning, I felt almost as helpless as the babies are. I had no idea what to do first. But it wasn't long until I had a tiny one in my own arms, bathing and giving routine morning care.

By the time the two of us took rectal temperatures, bathed, and diapered them all it was time to carry them out to their mothers to be fed. This morning the time just literally flew by. When I'm doing something I like, time always takes wings and flies away.

January 15, 1952: *Evening duty in the nursery is certainly a lot of fun. All we do between 7 and 9 p.m. is show the babies to the proud fathers, doting grandparents, solicitous uncles and aunts, curious cousins, friends, and any other interested parties. To watch the families' mixed emotions and expressions of love, adoration, surprise, and excitement surpasses any TV show.*

January 20, 1952 I soliloquized in another letter to Carl: *Wish you could peek at all my sweet, little darling babies. Sometimes they aren't so sweet, especially when one starts the solo recitative. Then the entire choir (a Capella, by the way) all join in forming a mighty chorus. As yet, it isn't too well balanced because some voices stick out above the others, but with a little practice and good leadership they should develop into a good, lusty chorale. They have a regular practice period and it's easy to tell what time it is about 1/2 hour before each meal. We usually take the loudest soloists (the ones who are hungriest) to their private eating places, their mothers. Then the rest of the chorus seems to be quieter by that time.*

However, hunger isn't the only stimulant for the lusty harmonies – they usually need dry pants now and then so they call individually for such a need. Also a slight tummy ache demands our undivided attention until they have burped satisfactorily. All in all, it's one very enjoyable cycle. Bye for now, M

January 28, 1952 Another long letter to Carl: *It is snowing big fat fleecy flakes here this afternoon, melting rapidly due to rain all forenoon, getting colder, and by morning it may be icy.*

Work in the delivery room (DR) is a grand adventure in itself. We were so dreadfully busy all day I didn't even realize it was Sunday. We weren't having any business in the DR the first part of my shift, so I was asked to help with the 20 babies in 3rd nursery.

It was so very hot and stuffy in there and, before I realized it, Megan, the graduate nurse working with me, groaned as she leaned against the table to balance herself. Then she just slumped to the floor – unconscious! I called for help and she soon revived but still felt woozy. The supervisor took her to the nurses' infirmary for a doctor to examine her and for her to recover completely. I bathed the babies and cleaned the nursery by myself. Later, we discovered she was pregnant.

All of a sudden things started happening again in the DR. I was called back there and another nurse took over the nursery. There were five admissions in the next four hours. From then on, we were so busy with four deliveries we hardly knew which end was up.

After all that frantic activity, I went off duty and raced several blocks to catch the bus to Mollie's home for some much needed rest and relaxation. Just as I got to the station, I watched the bus pull away. What a let-down. It's the first time I had ever missed it. So I waited for the 5:15 p.m. That didn't leave much time at home since I needed to be back by 10 p.m., but it was better than none at all.

Mollie's younger brother gave us a big laugh. In the course of our non-stop chatter, I commented that I would go to pediatrics (children's ward) to work after I'm finished on maternity.

Leslie said innocently, "Well, I thought you'd go there before eternity!" Just the way he said it made us hold our sides laughing. I still laugh when I think about it.

His twin sister was a little comedian, too. She caused us many tears of laughter by putting on an impromptu monologue of a radio program featuring the Jack Haynes show. Such a fun time we had that I came back to work well relaxed.

Caring for the mothers

February 15, 1952 My Journal speaks: *This week I worked 2nd floor postpartum on night duty. It wasn't quite as much fun taking care of the mothers as it was the babies. Mothers demanded attention about 3 or 4 a.m. when they should be sleeping. It amuses me how some of them are so utterly clueless when it comes to feeding their babies.*

For example, last night we took a baby out to her mother for the 2 a.m. feeding. A few minutes later she rang her bell. "My baby is sneezing. Is that serious?"

"Not at all," I replied in a reassuring voice. Not many minutes later she rang her bell again. "My baby has the hiccups, what should I do?"

By this time I was feeling a bit impatient. I thought to myself, anybody with a half teaspoon of common sense knows that hiccups are natural. I reassured her again, "Your little one is perfectly normal. Just feed her the way I showed you earlier."

Evidently my attempts to explain the process were in vain. Again she rang and said petulantly, "Would you come get my baby? I can't feed her any more. She just won't open her mouth."

The baby had only taken 1/2 ounce so I took her back to the nursery and within 10 minutes she had taken the whole two ounces. Some mothers are scared to death of their little cherubs. I think babies feel their mothers' insecurity and for that reason may not cooperate.

One mother begged the doctor to have the nurses feed her son in the nursery because she was scared she would drop him when she tried to burp him. Instead of alleviating her fears, the doctor gave us orders to feed him in the nursery and only show him to her once a day. That doctor was wrong, in my opinion. Why would anyone go through the whole nine-month pregnancy and not put forth more effort to learn about baby care ahead of time?

Marking halfway way point on maternity

February 28 marked the halfway point through my maternity rotation – my eighth week. Only two and a half weeks of night duty left. This siege of night duty was so much more enjoyable than the other times. Miss Rolle, the maternity night supervisor, was such a pleasant person. It was a pleasure to work under her. Also, the other staff people were easier to work with. I think bringing new life into the world created a more positive atmosphere and was such a welcome contrast to so much suffering and death in the other parts of the hospital.

A funny story

Adam Lapp, an Amish man, nervously paced the floor in the hallway waiting for news from the delivery room where his wife was giving birth. He anxiously watched me help another nurse quietly and skillfully transfer his sleepy wife, Mary, from the gurney to her hospital bed. He stroked his long beard streaked with gray as he greeted Mary. She had just given birth to a sweet baby girl, their tenth child, after a long, difficult labor and delivery due to complications during this pregnancy. This was the first time she gave birth in a hospital, and he was so worried about her that he hadn't slept for 20 hours.

After Mary was settled in her bed, he pulled out his pocket watch and saw that it was 3 a.m. There was no way he could go home 30 miles away at this hour. His brother had driven Adam and Mary to the hospital in his horse and buggy the day before and then returned home. Totally exhausted, he sat down heavily in the easy chair next to the bed.

The night light on the wall cast eerie shadows around the room. Every ten minutes I checked to make sure Mary wasn't hemorrhaging. Mr. Lapp woke up each time and apologized for being in my way. I reassured him that he was not a bother at all. On the fourth check, when I came into the darkened room and didn't see Mr. Lapp in the chair, I assumed he had stepped out of the room. After the fourth check, I knew Mary was in trouble. Her abdomen felt soft and spongy instead of firm as was expected after birth, and her blood pressure had plummeted precipitously. Mr. Lapp was nowhere to be seen, so I couldn't tell him what the situation was.

I hurried back to the nursing station with tremendous urgency to alert Miss R. that the lady needed medication to halt the hemorrhaging. Her hands were steady as she filled the syringe and raced back to the darkened room prepared to give Mary an intravenous medication by the light of the bedside nightlight. As she searched for the best vein on Mary's arm, she was totally unprepared for what happened next.

Just as she was ready to insert the needle into the vein, she saw in her peripheral vision two wide-open eyes, a hairy head, and scraggly beard slowly and quietly emerge from under the other side of the bed. It was Mr. Lapp wondering what was happening with his wife! His big questioning eyes looked around warily to see what all the commotion was about. He had decided to slip out of the chair and curl up under the bed on the cold hard tile floor to get out of our way.

Miss R. had no idea that a man was in the room. Shocked and frightened by this spectacle, she turned ghostly white and dropped the glass syringe with the medication. The syringe broke and the medicine splatted all over the floor. She exclaimed loudly, "Aye, Aye, Aye!" When she realized the hairy head was the patient's sleepy husband, she sheepishly apologized and returned to the nursing station to prepare another injection for the lady while I cleaned up the slippery mess on the floor.

The medicine soon took effect and the bleeding stopped, and I made my patient as comfortable as possible. Soon they were both sleeping peacefully, Mary in the bed and Adam in the chair again. I wondered what eerie graveyard shift adventures we would encounter next. We had to be prepared for anything because we never knew what to expect.

One night the police helped a mother deliver a healthy baby boy in the car on the way to the hospital. The baby and mother were both placed in a private room. It was a hospital policy to quarantine both mother and baby for 72 hours to make sure neither one had acquired an infection that could be transmitted to other patients.

March 2, 1952: *Last night, Wanda and I worked the night shift together in the delivery room. How could a place be so busy? From 12-5 a.m., we admitted eight patients at some stage of labor and delivered six babies by 7 a.m. Both delivery rooms were filled the whole time. As soon as one labor patient delivered, we wheeled her out quickly and another patient took her place. I kept very busy doing preps, giving medications, checking progression of the patients in the labor room to determine how close they were to delivery time, scrubbing for deliveries, and weighing the sweet babies after they were born.*

Oh yes, in between, when I had a few minutes, I gave progress reports to all the anxious fathers who were either pacing nervously in the hallway or sprawled out on the chairs in the waiting room trying to get a few winks of sleep.

The hubbub quieted down about 5:30 a.m., so I was asked to help Martha give bedpans to the post-partum patients on 3rd floor. It was more involved than just placing and removing a bedpan. At the same time we also gave perineum care to each patient by swabbing warm sterile water over a patient's perineum to prevent infection. So it took time to do all that, sometimes for as many as 22 patients.

[Author's note: In that era, newly delivered patients were not allowed out of bed to the bathroom for at least five days after delivery, thus the need to use bedpans.]

Next we went from delivering bedpans to feeding babies for the next hour. We were careful to wash our hands between each one, of course. Carol and I carried babies to their mothers for 6 a.m. feeding. We carried two at a time, one on each arm, since we weren't fortunate enough to have a cart to carry 8 or 10 at a time. We had to carefully check the ID bracelets to make sure we placed the right baby with the right mother.

After carrying 22 babies down those two long halls, we felt like we had run a marathon from here to San Francisco! By the time we did our charting we could hardly drag ourselves around another minute.

March 3, 1952: *At 3 a.m. after we fed babies and lulled them back to sleep, I began to feel drowsy myself and felt a pang of envy as I thought about my friends who would be snoozing peacefully in their cozy beds.*

Sitting on the hard, unforgiving chair at the nurses' station to do my charting, I wondered which mother would ring her bell next to ask for a pain pill, a bedpan, or just someone to talk to when she couldn't sleep.

Babies create a busy time in delivery rooms and nurseries

March 14, 1952: *This week I was assigned to work night shifts, part of that time in each of the two delivery rooms and on the three maternity floors that were even busier than last week.*

It's a long story, but here is a brief account of the struggles we've had:

It began to snow heavily around 10 p.m. Thursday night. Every pregnant woman in this county must have decided to go into labor and deliver her baby. Several of the women nearing their delivery date told us they were frightened at the prospect of being stranded by snow and unable to reach the hospital in time through blizzard conditions, so they decided to come in early. Can't say as I blame them for that. Between 12 and 5 a.m. we had 14 admissions, 4 deliveries, and 1 cesarean section!

The newborn babies just kept coming and coming into the nursery where I was working. I was so busy racing around the nursery, I hardly had time to breathe. Miss R. called in a couple of extra nurses to take my place and she asked me to go help in the delivery room since I had recent experience there.

When I got to the labor and delivery rooms the place was in a riotous uproar – patient charts were lying around everywhere and several patients were waiting on beds in the hallway, some in the labor rooms. We had to double and triple check to make sure that we charted the right things on the right patients' charts. This was just the last straw. How could we give good care under these stressful circumstances?

I scrubbed for a delivery at 6:50 a.m., consequently I didn't get off till 7:40. My legs were numb with fatigue. The poor doctors were nearly dead on their feet, too. One exhausted doctor sprawled out on a gurney and another curled up in a wheelchair in an attempt to catch a little sleep. Everyone was taxed to the very limit, physically and emotionally.

With all these deliveries in such a short time it turned out we did not have enough beds for them, so the orderlies went to the attic for extra beds to put in the hall. They also needed to get extra baby cribs. It was our job to clean all of them, too. No one had time to sit down for any kind of a break all night. Oh my! I don't know how we ever got through it. Mother Nature waits for no one.

Saturday night was worse yet. It was still snowing. We had seven more admissions and eight deliveries. Whoever heard of such a steady influx of patients? We were at our wits' end to know what to do with all of them. One lady in active labor had to lay on the gurney for nearly an hour before a bed in the labor room was available. Six more patients were on extra beds out in the hall, and one woman had to wait in the wheelchair until we could find her a bed. Not a good place to be for someone in active labor for more than an hour!

When 1st and 2nd floor rooms are filled up, patients are placed in 3rd floor rooms or in the hallway after they deliver their babies. Third floor maternity had a bed capacity for 22 patients but, by Sunday a.m., 31 were there.

Here's my latest escapade

April 10, 1952: *I had the unique opportunity to deliver a baby all by myself Saturday. The doctor didn't get there in time and there was another delivery going on in the other D.R. When I checked this patient, her baby was already on the way out. I managed to hold it back until we could get her over to the delivery table, then POP – the cutest little baby girl was born! It was quite a thrill. The evening duty* *supervisor was quite proud of "Dr. Minter" as she called me. Usually an intern or resident is there even if the patient's regular doctor isn't, but this time there was no one else available.*

We delivered 4 babies in 15 minutes...twins in one D.R, one in the other D.R. and one on the bed in the hall. Such a mess as we were in. Linens and sterile supplies were alarmingly low by that time. We didn't have enough help and all of us were at the point where we thought it couldn't get any worse, but somehow we all survived – how, I don't know. Obviously we weren't sitting around twiddling our thumbs.

April 15, 1952: *I added up the number of times that I scrubbed along with the doctors for deliveries. To my surprise, I had helped bring 52 babies into this cold world!*

This sinus infection and I have waged a personal civil war for a couple of days. We became antagonists on Friday evening when I thought it was warm enough to wear just a light jacket down town. With extra rest, forced fluids, and the good old standby "Vicks VapoRub" as my weapons, I will emerge the victorious conqueror.

More admissions

Every shift we admitted at least four new patients to the labor and delivery rooms. It was not a matter of merely saying, "Hello", either. Admitting a patient involved taking her vital signs (temperature, pulse, respiration, and blood pressure), timing her contractions, checking fetal heartbeats, and monitoring each patient's progress carefully during the labor process. After delivery, we checked for any post-partum hemorrhage.

When a post-partum patient was discharged to go home 7-10 days later, we sterilized the bed and side table, stripped the beds, and put on fresh linens. All this work was in addition to our other jobs. If my memory serves me right, we didn't have nurses' aides to help with the work. No wonder we were totally exhausted at the end of eight hour shifts.

April 20, 1952: *I ended my four months rotation on Maternity Ward with a sense of satisfaction and accomplishment mixed with awe and wonder at the whole idea of seeing new life emerge – innocent babies born with all their potential built into their tiny bodies, hearts and minds.*

Chapter 18
Pediatric Ward and Polio Unit

After that very long four month stretch of working nights and evenings on maternity, it was strange to work a day shift again. Pediatric Ward was a totally different, but heart-warming experience – working with sick children for five weeks. All but two of the 11 patients were ambulatory and out of bed, so we didn't have as much bedside care.

April 29, 1952: *Would you enjoy a bird's eye view into Kids' Ward for just a few moments? Today was my first day on Pediatric Ward. Already my mind has been opened to new vistas of learning, and it has added to my knowledge of children. Such darling ones we have up there! I thoroughly enjoyed maternity, but Kids Ward is even better, if that's possible. I can put my heart and soul into my work as never before…working with small children…alleviating their distresses…listening to their problems…reassuring them by a squeeze of their little hands that everything will work out OK…quieting a child's fears. All this and more gives me such a sense of utter satisfaction that nothing else has accomplished up to now.*

Four-year-old Leroy pulls on my heartstrings more than anyone else. He is the unfortunate victim of the dreaded enemy, cancer. It has spread to his lungs, giving him NO chance of survival because it has left him with a minimum of healthy lung tissue. To watch him suffer…gasp for that precious breath of life…see him slowly being suffocated by the malignant growth…to know there is absolutely nothing more that we can do to alleviate his discomfort, it nearly breaks my heart to see a sweet little life being gradually snuffed out like that. In one way I look at it, watching an old person die is easier than watching a child die gasping for breath.

Ten-year-old Sandra is an only child who is stubborn and spoiled. She is quite a problem when it comes to taking her medication. She sulks, kicks and sometimes screams – a very unladylike custom for her age. My heart aches for her too. She confided to me her longing, the soul hunger she has had for the companionship of a father. She was six months old when her father divorced her mother. He lives in another city now. Not having known the love of a dear father must leave a great vacancy in a young person's life.

Nine year old Patsy is slowly recovering from the removal of a nearly ruptured appendix. She is very sick and it gives pleasure to both of us when I even so much as refill the ice pack to place on her feverish brow. She calls me "my nurse."

Terry calls from the bed in the corner, "Nurse!" I know that he is going to ask in a pitiful, plaintive voice that melts my heart, "When are my mommy and daddy coming to see me?"

Each child has their own special personality to deal with. My understanding of children's problems, fears, and moods has been broadened considerably. It challenges the very deepest maternal instinct within each of us nurses to show these youngsters all the love and understanding we can. Some have gotten more love in here than they get at home. And so it goes. Each one of our 25 patients – little or big – demands all the tactful nursing skill and patience that we can give. This morning as we were giving baths we laughed a lot as young Harold highly entertained us by reading moron jokes out loud to us as we worked.

A day at the beach

One summer morning, after finishing our night shift on Pediatrics, four of us nurses hatched the brainy idea to spend the day at the beach near Ocean City, New Jersey, two hours away. We dabbled our feet in the cool water and allowed the waves to wash over us before we spread our towels on the sand and ate our picnic lunch in the bright noonday sun. We alternated splashing in the surf and sun-bathing the rest of the afternoon. I stretched out on my beach towel and tried to catch a few ZZZZs while listening to the roar of the vast ocean as the surf crashed on the shore.

It was blissful to allow the sun's warmth to relax my tired body after having worked all night. It felt so good – at first. I didn't realize just how long I laid there and how hot the sun was, though. By mid-afternoon, my back, neck, arms, and legs were fiery red and extremely painful. My sunburned skin felt like I was on fire, and I could hardly walk upright. How naïve I was having had minimal experience at the beach. I had soaked up too much sun too fast. It wasn't so blissful then. I realized how lying in the midday sun carried devastating consequences.

We returned about 6:15 that evening having had precious little sleep all day. I barely managed to sleep two more hours before I went to work at 11 p.m. That night on duty, my starched, scratchy uniform magnified the pain from the sunburn. Ouch!

I had a terrible time staying awake, too. Somehow I made it through those eight excruciating hours of night shift. I learned an important lesson about the intensity of sunbathing in the midday sun, and I felt the effects for several days.

May 18, 1952: *On Kids' Ward, our time is spent feeding the youngest ones, spoiling them, playing games, and reading stories to them. Doesn't feel like work at all. It was quiet this evening because we had no critically ill patients. I don't particularly like to work with Dottie, though. She is too rough and very bossy with the children.*

May 22, 1952: *Tonight was busier than usual. We admitted two very sick children after 7 pm. Several youngsters decided to be contrary. Three-year-old Marlene had a streak of screaming until 9 pm. I rubbed her tummy gently and soon she quieted down and went to sleep. Some children need more touch/attention than others.*

Billy became stubborn, too, and wouldn't eat his supper. Soon three of the babies started yelling at the same time. It was one grand cacophony of noise in addition to visitors coming and going. By 9:45 we were nearly at our wits' end, but the children had quieted down by the time we went home at 11:30 p.m.

June 16, 1952: *Long summer days are unbearably HOT. Patty and I gulped copious quantities of iced tea as we worked with the children. When I have a split shift, instead of eating dinner I often sleep on my mid-day hours off – 11-3:30 – because I am dead tired from lack of sleep.*

The next two-week stretch I am scheduled for what is called PRN, which means the supervisor schedules me on different shifts and wards wherever she needs an extra nurse. In my opinion, it is the most fatiguing and unforgiving business ever. Being assigned to a different ward with patients I don't know can be so frustrating. I'll be glad when the two weeks are over. This must be preparing us for what the REAL world of nursing is like. Hmmm! I better get used to it.

June 23, 1952: *Tonight I'm on evening duty and am scheduled to work a day shift tomorrow which means I have to sleep fast when I get off duty. It's really rugged doing what we call "double back" shifts: off duty at 7:30 a.m., back to work at 3 till 11:30 p.m., and on duty again the next morning at 7 a.m. I think the powers that be want to see how hard they can push us physically and emotionally. Oh well, enough complaining, Minnie.*

June 26, 1952: *We had two youngsters who needed tepid sponge baths to lower their high body temperatures. All the kids were irritable because the heat and humidity were intense and unbearably stifling. I pitied them because it was too hot to even think of sleeping.*

Four-year-old Paul Henry wanted to say his prayers tonight, so I helped him say "Now I lay me down to sleep." Then I asked him if he ever heard about Jesus. He said no, he hadn't. So I told him the whole story, then he asked me to tell it again, and then still a third time. "Let the little children come unto me," said Jesus.

After I was off duty, I had a terrible time going to sleep. It was simply a sauna-bake-oven temperature. The radio said it was the hottest day in 80 years.

June 29, 1952: *This was another difficult night shift not only did I fight to stay awake, but we admitted a little curly-haired baby girl, six months old with dehydration and heat prostration. Berta was her special nurse all night. She was in an oxygen tent with plasma and glucose IV by venesection. We tepid-sponged her for a body temperature of 108. We wanted her to live so badly, but she died early this morning. It was really sad. She was such a sweet little girl.*

July 2, 1952: *The new interns started their year of internship yesterday. They are such cute guys. They remind me of when we were probies. They didn't know what to do or how to go ahead. Dr. Holman is working here on Pediatrics.*

Miss. B. gave me 90 in my efficiency evaluation on pediatrics. I was real tickled about that. She also told me that I was to be transferred to the Polio Ward for two weeks. That would be an interesting change. Only one patient is there now.

Breaking my heart

This is a peek into my journal about the emotional trauma I went through when Carl decided to break up our relationship during my time in the Pediatric Ward.

May 7, 1952: *Last week when I spent the day at the college on my day off, I felt some tension when Carl and I had some time together. I had a vague feeling that all was not right between us, but I couldn't tell what it was. It was a strange sensation of not knowing what to expect. He seemed to be terribly uptight about something, not relaxed like he usually was. After supper, we went for a walk on the trail and sat down on the little bench fastened between two trees.*

He talked about his spiritual problems and how he feels in need of revival. He said he feels his soul is lean. He acknowledged, that among other things, his lack of ability to delegate tasks led to compulsive overwork as the yearbook editor and it has contributed to his spiritual lethargy as well as the cooling of our relationship.

I was completely taken off balance by what he said next. He says he is very confused about our relationship and doesn't think he loves me to the extent that I love him...doesn't think that we'd be good life companions. But yet he told me three times while sitting there that he loves me. He said he was sorry for hurting me. Well, that only made me feel worse. If he is so sorry why was he doing this? What confusing, mixed messages!

I began to feel angry. This person who has called me his sweetheart for the last two years and led me to believe that he wanted us to be life companions was suddenly flaunting rejection in my face. He said he was breaking up our courtship for an indefinite period of time. Oh, what a crushing, confusing blow this was to me! We drove in silence on the way back to the hospital. There was nothing more to say.

The next few days, I felt like the very life was being squeezed out of my being. I felt like screaming much of the time. But God's promise to strengthen me was a comforting thought that I hung on to for dear life. I knew He would stand by me faithfully. Oh, it was hard. Terribly hard!

In the weeks that followed, the time dragged by oh so slowly. I went about my work as usual, but with very little enthusiasm. I couldn't help but wonder if it was something I had done that changed his mind, but I couldn't come up with anything.

June 10, 1952: *A whole month has passed, and here it is Friday night – a date night for us, Carl and I, often. There would be no date tonight. A great loneliness and sadness came over me like a big black cloud that I couldn't shake off. When I knelt to pray, the vision of our parting came over me with such force I ended up crying almost hysterically for a long time. It's been over a month since I've heard from him, and the time goes so slow. Will we ever see each other again? Perhaps never. I must accept this and move on.*

"My thoughts are not your thoughts, neither are my ways your ways, thus saith the Lord." Maybe He has something better in mind for me. It's wonderful to trust in Him, but I don't do it well enough.

I ordered one of the college yearbooks that Carl has worked on so hard this past school year. Even though his hard work on it contributed to our breakup, I will still treasure it for years to come.

[The first week in July, after his semester tests and difficult work on the yearbook were over, he called me and asked if we could try to patch things up. I wasn't sure if I could trust him. I still had doubts and questions. Was he just jerking me around emotionally? He said he had worked through his doubts and wanted to pick up the relationship where we left off. He also said he wanted to continue our plans to drive together to my parents' home in Kansas for my vacation in August. He came to see me later that week, and we were able to talk out some of our feelings. I felt some relief from the oppressive feelings.]

Beginning Polio Unit

July 10, 1952: *My first day on the Polio Unit was fascinating to say the least…totally different than any other type of nursing that I've done so far. We have only one patient, an 11-year old girl, Mari Alice. She is in isolation because polio is very contagious. That means we have to wear gown, gloves, and mask, and go through elaborate sterile procedures (similar to when I worked in surgery) before and after we work with her.*

She's a brave little person. Nursing care involves laying hot moist packs on both of her legs six times a day. Both of her legs are paralyzed, one is more paralyzed than the other. We use what is called the Kenny Packer. The moist compresses relax the affected muscles, followed by passive exercises, gentle massage, and/or hydrotherapy (warm baths) designed to restore function of the paralyzed muscles.

July 11, 1952: *Evening duty – we admitted Marty Lou, another polio patient, 15-years-old and so cute but very spoiled. Now she has four nurses to care for her and spoil her even more. She has a dramatic sense of humor, is very mature and well-informed for her age, and keeps us entertained by her antics.*

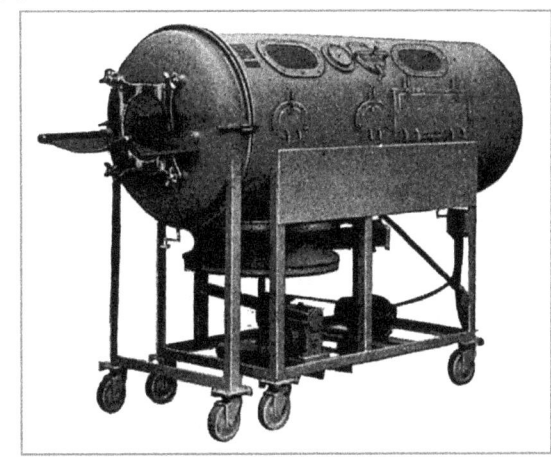

Her breathing muscles were affected and she's likely to contract pneumonia, aspirate secretions, or suffocate. We placed her in what is called an iron lung, a massive machine that will

maintain her respiration artificially until she can breathe on her own. [Today we would call it a respirator.]

It is powered by an electric motor and pulls air in and out of the lungs by changing the pressure inside the machine. I don't understand all of it, but that's how it was explained to me. Her leg muscles aren't completely paralyzed, but they do not react the way normal muscles should so we use the hot moist packs with her, too. She is to be transferred to another hospital tomorrow where she can get more respiratory support.

Her mother, an organist at Mt. Calvary Lutheran Church, said she would give me organ lessons free if I want them. Her father is manager of some big corporation. They are quite "ritzy."

It is hard for four people to look busy with just two patients, even though each patient needs lots of nursing care. More victims of this dreaded disease will probably come in as the polio season progresses.

Anticipating vacation

July 14, 1952: *History has another day to its credit, and I am glad, glad, glad. This will be a long, boring week. I'm so eager for my vacation to start Friday when Carl and I are leaving for my home in Kansas. Imagine! Four weeks away from this stifling, hot hospital. On second thought, Kansas will probably be hot, also.*

Mrs. Rueben, the nurses' aide on the Polio Unit, has been telling me her story about her life in a concentration camp in Latvia during WW2. She and part of her family spent 3 years in a German concentration camp. It just makes my heart bleed to think of all she went through…starvation, hard physical labor, physical and mental abuse. Here, we grumble and complain about trivial and trifling things. I could kick myself for doing that.

July 16, 1952: *Today was terribly monotonous on Polio because Mari Alice is out of isolation now, and we only have to put hot wet packs on her legs four times a day. That means even less for us to do. She is improving rapidly and was able to be out in the chair today. To* *celebrate her coming out of isolation, we had a party of ice cream, potato chips, and pretzels with iced tea.*

July 17, 1952: *I can hardly stand how slow these days are going, especially since we have only one patient to care for now. God willing, this time tomorrow night Carl and I will be on our way to Kansas to see my family. I get goosebumps and can hardly wait!*

Working on the Pediatric and Polio Wards has been enjoyable for me – slower pace and less pressure. Since I'm going away for four weeks on vacation, I will never know how each of the patients progressed in their recovery. They will have been discharged and gone home before I return.

Tonight my dear friend Mollie begins her first stint of night duty on Women's Medical Ward. I sure hope it goes well for her. Anything can happen there, from Granny falling out of bed and breaking her hip to a suicidal patient trying to cut her wrists with the glass drinking straw that she broke in half. That really has happened, believe me!

Vacation time

Between July 20 and August 22, Carl and I enjoyed our vacation trip to visit my parents, siblings, and friends in Kansas. Mollie's 12-year-old twin siblings also went with us and provided us with comedy and laughter.

The first three weeks we helped a neighbor paint the exterior of his house, enjoyed picnics in the park, had fun family times around the kitchen table, and provided the music for a friend's wedding. We also went to Oklahoma for a few days to visit relatives I hadn't seen in a long time.

The beginning of the fourth week we said goodbye to my family and drove to a mission station in Kentucky where Carl was scheduled to be the minister for two weeks of evangelistic tent meetings with two of his college preacher-friends.

Impressions of Kentucky: *Kentucky was beautiful at that time of the year. It was interesting to get to know various people there and their unique ways of living. I wish I could write all the impressions I received such as the true country singing, mothers informally breast feeding babies in church, their honeyed speech and soft-flowing accent that drawls so pleasantly. They come to church one half to one hour early because they have no clocks – they just sit and frankly stare unabashedly at us as strangers; the men congregate and idle away their days chewing and spitting tobacco as they exchange the latest community gossip; the large families; their easy-going way of life; the rocky, rutty and almost impassable "roads" – really only paths – but the Chevy got through! I spent time reading my book, The Enduring Hills, that portrays the life of the Kentucky people.*

After goodbyes to Carl, the twins and I drove back to PA without any car trouble.

Chapter 19
Back to Work at LGH

An erratic schedule/moving to the new wing

August 22, 1952: *This was an ordinary workday with a split-shift on Women's Surgical at LGH after a wonderful month of vacation. I slept during most of my time off this afternoon. It's nice to just have time to relax after that long car trip.*

August 24, 1952: *Miss R. sent me over to help on 3rd floor maternity this morning. We were frightfully busy. It is always a mad house there when patients are popping babies out right and left. I was the only student there after 12:30. After doing five discharges, I was so weary I almost felt sick when I went off duty at 3:30. Ah me! I'm still recovering from the vacation road trip that just ended, I guess.*

August 28, 1952: *What a day this has been – the office changed our schedules all around and that put everyone in a foul mood. I'm scheduled to work day duty this coming week.*

When Miss R. took away Doris' Sunday off, Doris said angrily, "I'm quitting!" All of us were on edge and wondered if our days off would be taken away, too. Later the supervisor relented, reconfigured the schedule, and allowed Doris to have her Sunday off. Doris finally calmed down.

The latest news around here is that we're getting ready to move patients, equipment, and supplies to the new hospital addition. That should be interesting.

August 30, 1952: *At 8 a.m., Miss R. got a call that Mrs. Hilt wouldn't be coming in for evening duty the next two nights. Guess who was asked to work till 11 a.m. with time off between 11-7 and then work 7-11 p.m.? That's right, yours truly. I hardly knew what to do with myself all day. I decided this was a good time to read the book assignment "Asylum" to prepare for my psychiatric rotation at Byberry State Hospital that starts next Sunday.*

August 31, 1952: *Last night my patient Mrs. Komis, who says she's of the Greek Orthodox religion, came up with the crazy idea that she was going to die. I spent 15 minutes listening to her, and she insisted she was ready to die.*

Another patient, Maggie R. got a phone call from her boyfriend in Austin, Texas. Since there are no bedside telephones, I moved her bed out into the hall as far as I could so she could talk to him on the telephone in the nurses' station.

I found out I'm scheduled to go on day duty tomorrow instead of evening duty. I really don't know what's going on or what I'm supposed to be doing. Our hours get changed around so much without notifying us until the very last minute. I feel like I am just a pawn in a roulette game or something.

September 1, 1952: *Believe it or not, today we started the process of moving supplies from Women's Surgical to 3rd East Wing in the new part of the hospital. That's the latest excitement around here. Tomorrow we will move patients and all their personal belongings and leave the old furniture and equipment behind. Brand new furniture and equipment are waiting for us there. It will be wonderful to work with new stuff in a shiny new building. Construction has been so slow; I thought I'd never actually see the day that I would work there.*

September 3, 1952: *I'm relaxing to beautiful concert music as I write. What momentous historic two days these have been as we plunged ourselves deeper into the heat of moving this morning. It was a big job moving everything in addition to caring for the patients. They all cooperated very well, so it didn't seem to be too traumatic for them.*

By 1:30 p.m. we had transferred all twenty patients from Women's Surgical Ward to 3rd East Wing in the beautiful new part of the hospital. There are sixteen private rooms and four double rooms with a long hall. We hardly know how to act over there with everything brand new, sparkling clean, and very convenient. I'm sure we will run our poor legs off up and down the long halls. The new intercom call system is fun to use and will save us nurses a lot of steps.

September 4, 1952: *I was happily working with surgical patients on 3rd East when I was again asked to go and work in Preemie Nursery on Maternity Wing. I don't much like to work with preemies (they are so fragile), but I stayed till 3:30 anyway. Just another vivid example of how we get jerked around with very little notice whether we want to or not.*

September 5, 1952: *This has been a good day – I'm happy and contented for a change – eager for whatever might be waiting for me. Who knows how long that contentment will last? Working in a brand new building with mostly private rooms has lifted my spirits, I think.*

Mr. Haven was one of my patients. He's a mess with his bloody, broken nose, bad breath, and voiding involuntarily. Two of my patients, a man and his wife, are in the same double room and we joke a lot with each other.

Now I must get to bed or I'll never get up in time for a special morning chapel tomorrow.

Part Four

One Year as Senior Students

Chapter 20
Second Black Velvet Band for Our Caps

Our second black band; strutting again!

September 11, 1952: *Congratulations, Minnie! You've become a senior today. How thrilling to finally be full-fledged SENIORS. We were officially declared seniors by the honorable Mrs. K. herself as she gave each of us our second coveted black velvet ribbon to add to the one we attached to our caps last year at this time. It is such a great feeling to wear my student cap with the two black bands. This day seemed ever so far away 2 years ago.*

And then, do we ever strut again! Feelings of elation, ecstasy, and dignity filled our hearts to think we really have become seniors. It was amazing what a difference it makes to have not just one but two black bands on our caps. The doctors and nursing supervisors actually treat us with even more respect – like we are human beings -- and consider that we might have some sense after all.

What will it be like when we become graduates? Will our heads actually swell? Oh well, that's another whole year away. And yet it will creep up stealthily before we realize it.

This was quite a busy day – 3rd East is really getting lively after we admitted several new patients. Now that we have nearly all private rooms, we do much more walking than we ever did in the older part of the hospital where patients were all in one large ward. The intercom is handy and helps to save our energies. If the patient calls in to the nurses' station for something, he/she can tell us over the intercom and we don't have to first make a trip to that room to find out what is needed. Oh, the wonders of technology.

September 12, 1952: *Another day has come and gone – life is like a vapor which we see for a moment and then we see it no more. It was busy on evening duty tonight but nothing like 2nd East was – they now have 31 patients.*

Groan! I must double back for day duty early tomorrow. I will have 3 pre-op patients to give skin preps and enemas to get ready for early surgery. That means I'll be extra busy. So I better get to bed.

September 13, 1952: *We went around in circles all day today. One of our post-ops went into shock...so many IVs to start...doctors making rounds...everything happening at once. I was so ready to leave at 3:30.*

I still had to rush around to change clothes so I could attend Wanda and Harry's wedding which was to start at 4 o'clock. Naomi and I dashed to the church, and we barely made it in time.

What a splashy affair! Wanda was a lovely bride with four bridesmaids and a maid of honor. Their dresses were simply beautiful. It was a long ceremony with communion at the altar. I talked to Dave and Marla afterwards. Their wedding is next Saturday. I wish Carl and I could get married like all our friends are doing. It must be wonderful...Sigh. Maybe sometime it will be our turn.

September 14, 1952: *This has been quite the day. It was such a relief to get off duty, and even then I was most too tired to do anything but flop on my bed and groan. I thought I'd simply die of fatigue. Mrs. S. and I were the only nurses on duty from 12-3:30. I had to prepare three patients for immediate surgery – 3 catheterizations and 3 enemas. I had trouble finding all the supplies I needed since we moved over here so recently. It was nerve-wracking, to say the least.*

September 15, 1952: *Viola, the nurses' aide, and I were very busy tonight. She was a dear and baked an apple pie for me. Bless her heart. Something to share with my dorm buddies later.*

All of the new rooms are now occupied, and it can get chaotic very fast. We have five demanding patients. They strike me as being so spoiled; I'd like to tell a few of them a thing or two, but since they have money for private rooms we must cater to their whims.

Mr. Oliver pouted all night because Dr. E. wouldn't let him go home for his Jewish holiday celebrations. Mrs. H. and Mrs. C. are two of a kind in the same room. Both are very demanding. Mrs. Z. wanted a snack in the middle of my shift so I stopped what I was doing to fix that for her. Mrs. M. was incontinent and needed bed linen changed – twice.

September 18, 1952: *Tonight Mr. Oliver was still pouting, and Mrs. C. screamed, "I want my water taken. You'll have to tap me!" So I catheterized her as soon as I could. I try hard to keep calm, collected and not become irritable, but some patients try my patience to the utmost! (Pun intended)*

After a night like tonight, I could throw my hands up in dismay and wonder why I ever wanted to be a nurse. But wait – nursing has brighter aspects – some nice, congenial, cheerful people boost our morale.

Here in the new part of the hospital we get the "cream of society." Ritzy big shots are used to everything being deluxe. We try hard to please everybody, but with 23 or more patients to care for, one or two nurses can only do so much. I want to keep the Golden Rule in mind when I care for patients: Treat them like I would want to be treated if I'm hurting.

September 19, 1952: *I'm fine and dandy and feel good tonight for three reasons:*

1) *I finished my pediatric case study today and got that load off my chest. I hated to start it, but am so glad it's finished.*

2) *Mrs. M. was so sweet to give me a chantilly perfume stick. I've always liked that fragrance.*

3) *I received a good letter from Carl today that boosted my spirits a lot. He's back in school loaded up with studies again.*

Mrs. C. had surgery for a nailed hip and really gave us a scare by reacting to medication. Her respirations decreased, blood pressure plummeted, pulse raced. We thought we would lose her, but the doctor was there and was able to give an antidote.

Mr. Oliver was over his pouting. He is a dear and cooperated tonight for a change. Our patients must be feeling better – they are more agreeable now, so that's something very different. Maybe the patients were sensing our anxiety over the newness of moving to the new wing. Or could it be I've had an attitude adjustment? Yes, that must be what makes the difference.

Chapter 21
Psychiatric Rotation

In the middle of September, Mrs. K. gave the spending money and textbooks to our group of 18 seniors as we were set to begin our three-month psychiatric rotation at Philadelphia State Hospital - Byberry. I packed my two suitcases – one big one and one small one – did laundry, and finished my required reading assignment *Asylum*. It was a creepy book about life in a mental hospital, supposedly to prepare me for this next rotation. If my experience even was to come close to what the book describes, it would be a wild ride.

Arriving at the State Hospital

September 21, 1952: *This is the day, the time, and the place that I've been anticipating with mixed feelings – Byberry! Dave's parents offered to take me along to Philadelphia when they took him to the university. They dropped me off at the nurses' residence and Dave was in such a big hurry he grabbed a suitcase, brought it to my room, and left right away. After they left, to my utter dismay, I discovered he only brought my small suitcase and left my big suitcase in their car. I was frantic. How in the world was I going to get on without it?! A sinking feeling came over me. I had no idea how to contact Dave or his parents in that big city. In my frustration, I prayed God would help me find it tomorrow. That put my mind at ease – for now anyway.*

The other girls heard about my predicament and offered to loan me what I needed for tonight and tomorrow: pajamas, a uniform, and shoes. I had my toiletries with me in my smaller suitcase. I have faith that the Lord will work things out, and I trust whoever unloads Dave's stuff will see my suitcase and leave it in a secure place. I can't do anything about it until tomorrow.

How do I feel right now at this very foreign-feeling huge State Hospital? Lost. My suitcase is missing! I am in a totally strange place with lots of unfamiliar faces. I must not panic, take it a step at a time and everything will be O.K. Take some deep breaths.

Getting acquainted

We were a group of 46 student nurses from nine different area hospitals, 18 of us from LGH. Most were very friendly. I was happy to find out we were settled into a modern and pleasant nurses' residence with private rooms and baths. There was a house mother on duty all the time. The regulations were pretty stiff. We had to sign in and out even to go to the mail box and back. We were advised that we should never walk anywhere on the grounds alone, but always in a group. I'm sure that was for our protection.

The brochure told us the Byberry campus covered 1,185 acres, including 500 acres of farm land and an undetermined number of formidable gray concrete buildings where the patients lived. The buildings all looked alike and resembled huge warehouses three and four stories high. More than 6,350 patients lived in those buildings. It was a small city in itself, enclosed with a secured high metal fence. It was simply immense. Totally awesome.

September 22, 1952: *None of us slept very well last night. Periodically blood-curdling screams pierced the long night silence. They were from the buildings across the street where patients are housed. We are tense and on edge with apprehension wondering what is in store for us. This is a whole new ballgame we're getting into.*

Today's agenda included general information and orientation, a psychology lecture, dinner, another lecture on general management of patients, and a tour of several buildings.

Miss B. issued each student a 4 ½ foot long link chain with a heavy brass ring at the end. On the ring were 16 keys – a key for each building, I would guess. The key ring also holds a police whistle if I need to summon help at any time. I fastened the chain around my waist and dropped the keys in my uniform pocket where they make a big bulge under my apron and jangle as I walk. I feel like a jailer. Every door in this huge complex is securely locked so we must know which key to use. It will take time to master that skill.

At 3 o'clock we were dismissed, so it was time to bravely start out to find my suitcase. I first called Angie at the Mission to see how to contact the Smiths where Dave was supposed to be staying. I was told they do not have a phone, so Angie suggested I call Anna. When I finally got through to her, we arranged to meet at the Jefferson Hospital where she works in downtown Philly. I dreaded going into the big city on faith alone by myself, not knowing whether my suitcase would be there, but I couldn't think of any other way to get it.

Bless their hearts, Jean, Patty, Riley, and Rita offered to go with me, and together we bravely faced the formidable public transportation system in that huge city. Byberry State Hospital is located at the northeast edge approximately 20 miles from city center. What an epic adventure for a farm girl from Kansas.

With the help of a city map and Anna's good directions, we made connections. It wasn't as complicated as we thought it might be. We arrived at Smith's home and—joy of joys – there was my suitcase! I could have kissed that battered old suitcase. What a relief. I was one happy camper.

Now after traveling on the trolley and the bus 1½ hours one way we are back at our nurses' residence. We celebrated our success by eating the food Carl's mother sent with me. I returned the things that my friends so kindly loaned me and felt very grateful. This has been a day I'll never forget as long as my memory proves true to me.

Oh yes, today is Carl's 21st birthday. Hope he had a happy day.

(During the months I was at Byberry, I rode the bus or train to Elizabethtown several weekends and he came to visit me twice while I was there.)

September 23, 1952: *This place gets more interesting each day. The dining room for the student nurses is quite unique. In the center of the room is a big square food bar loaded with every imaginable kind of fruits and vegetables that make wonderful salads. I'm sure we'll be well fed.*

Three classes, a film on hydrotherapy, and a tour through three buildings made up our day. We will work mostly all day duty shifts and have most weekends off. That will be a nice change. I don't know what there is to do on Sundays yet. Trust me, I'll find something fun to do.

September 24, 1952: *This has been a rare day. We were so restless in the two classes that we could hardly sit any longer. Miss P took us on a long tour through more buildings: the tuberculosis patient ward and the wards across the boulevard where men are housed. All of them smelled terrible. How anyone can work in that stench is beyond me. I guess I'm about to find out. Some of the inmates look pathetic. It's hard to understand how a human being can get that low.*

After the evening meal, Riley suggested a few of us walk over to the administration building and watch the patients dance. Riley, Patty, Norma, and I were standing in a clump together when this handsome young fellow named Freddy walked up to us. I was surprised when he singled me out. He asked my name and then saw my prayer-covering which I wore when I wasn't on duty.

He began to rave over me: "You are SO pretty and I can hardly wait to dance with you." He talked about the plain girls (Mennonite) who were here with the last group of students from LGH – Ettie, Hallie, and Greta.

Freddy's comment was, "Ettie had the brains but no love, and she wore dresses like the Pilgrims brought over on the Mayflower. Her great-grandmother packed them away in mothballs for 300 years."

He expounded further: "Hallie's eyes were so beautiful I could look into them forever. I fall in love with all the Mennonite girls. I'm going to join the Mennonite church someday so I can date their girls." I had such a hard time to keep from laughing in his face. I laughed on the inside, though.

Freddy also rattled on and on about a female patient he had danced with earlier. She had asked him, "Did you bring the engagement ring with you? Or, did you leave it at the house?" "Yes, I left it at the house," he stammered, glad for an excuse to lean on.

The Jewish man was preaching to Patty from his Hebrew Bible. A little old lady sang her incomprehensible song over the microphone and when she was finished she yelled, "Well, come on, clap everybody. WAKE UP."

So we clapped politely. At 7:30 the four of us walked back to our residence. When I told Sallie about Freddy, I thought she would simply pass out with laughter.

Starting classes

September 25, 1952: *We are sitting in a boring 2 hour lecture by Dr. H. on the History and objectives of psychiatry. Now, I'm not interested in what Napoleon or Mussolini thought any more than I am interested in whether the cat killed the mouse. It's such a dry subject. In fact, the instructor placed a pitcher of water and a glass on the doctor's desk. When the class period was over the water pitcher was almost empty. Now that's dry.*

This is our last day of all-day classes. Tomorrow we start on the wards and will have only one class a day. Today the lesson was on how to deal with violent patients. They taught us the techniques of releasing a patient's grasp on our hair, how to get a patient to walk when he or she stubbornly refuses, how to protect ourselves if a patient attacks us with a knife or throws objects at us. I shiver to think of meeting up with such a situation. I'll be petrified if that ever happens.

Starting to work with patients

My group's first taste of working on N-3 Ward was pretty scary. The big room had 65 single cots lined up in rows for female patients from ages 19-35 years old. All have histories of violence. Ten of them were shackled, strapped down with cuffs and straps by their wrists and ankles in their beds so they couldn't act out violently.

One patient worked herself out of the straps in some ingenious way. Before we knew it she had pushed out a window pane and crawled out over the door transom. Her wrist and arm were badly slashed and they had to take her for treatment. Breaking windows was their favorite hobby, we were told. Some patients' arms and wrists were terribly scarred.

There were only three male attendants and two female attendants who mainly stood around passively, it seemed to us. They were vigilant, but in my opinion, there should have been more of them for that many patients. They were there mainly to make sure the women didn't kill themselves or each other.

Every new admission had to be carefully searched for contraband items. All incoming and outgoing mail was censored. We closely supervised anyone smoking to prevent setting a fire.

September 27, 1952: *This was the first weekend we were required to work. Several of us were again assigned to 3rd floor of N3 yesterday. Our knees were shaking to think of what might be waiting there for us. Six patients were in restraints and four of those were locked in seclusion. In the dayroom, others assaulted us verbally.*

Anna really got angry one time and stomped around shouting obscenities, so we put her in seclusion. Irene became violent over some perceived minor incident. She started throwing things, so we restrained her. Lucy screamed and carried on something terrible. It took eight of us to hold her down while we put her in cuffs. We tried to reason with them in a moderate tone of voice, but that seemed to aggravate them even more.

Two teenagers, Dorothy and Elizabeth, are in seclusion. They are just plain bad girls. Together they broke 31 windows the first night they came in, we were told. They also said they'll kill us all if they get the chance. I'll bet they would, too, no doubt about it. I wouldn't want to meet them in a dark alley.

After all that morning activity, we finally organized ourselves and were ready to give patients oral hygiene, supervise smoking, and make sure they all showered, (such smelly people!).

Several women were scheduled for electro-convulsive shock therapy (ECT). My job was to help give ECT to three patients. What a day this has been. Now I'm wiser, warier, and weaker because this kind of work emotionally drains me.

Tonight we set our clocks back an hour to give us an extra hour of sleep. That will be refreshing. Now I must get to bed so I can get up tomorrow morning without feeling like a sick puppy. I'm so tired I think I'll flop on my bed like a rag doll.

Let me give a brief description of how electro-convulsive therapy was used at this time on patients with major depression. I used leather straps to secure the patient on a stretcher and placed electrodes on each side of the head over each temple. Next, I placed a soft rubber tube in her mouth for her to bite down on. This prevented her from biting her lips and tongue when she clamped her jaws down hard during the convulsions.

The doctor then turned on electrical current that went through the electrodes to her brain. She reacted by going into severe epileptic-type grand mal convulsions for about one and a half minutes. It was not a pretty sight to watch someone seize and foam at the mouth. She was unconscious and felt no pain at that point. When the convulsions stopped, she was dazed and disoriented for a few minutes but gradually returned to consciousness and we took her back to her bed. The goal of daily ECT was to produce a certain level of forgetfulness of what caused the patient to be depressed in the first place. Over time, her mental condition gradually improved.

[Currently ECT is done in a much more humane manner. A muscle relaxant is injected intramuscularly prior to the procedure that reduces seizures to minimal activity (only the toes wiggle during the procedure) but still results in a certain level of amnesia. A fuller explanation of the procedure can be found at www.hopkinsmedicine.org/psychiatry/specialty_areas/brain]

September 29, 1952, Patient admission day: *This turned out to be quite a frustrating day. First of all, my student group was frustrated with the two supervisors. They don't seem to know how to delegate tasks most of the time. Nothing seems to be organized. Six new patients came to our ward. That meant each one has to be showered, de-*

loused, vital signs taken, given an enema, and then have an interview with the psychiatrist.

What a job it is to make sure everyone showers and shampoos properly and then to select the clothes that fit them. Lucy's dress has buttons missing; Dorothy's stockings don't match; Mabel's slip sticks out 4 inches; Isabelle and Anna are fighting over who gets to use the bathtub first.

Three of the admissions were girls 15, 16, and 20 years old. Beth was very violent, so we put her in restraints right away; Helen cussed up a storm of profanity like my ears have never heard before. Others were totally confused about where they were. Rose was delusional as she stood in the hallway repeatedly yelling at us, "I'm talking to the man next door."

When I approached her, she assured me, "I'm not crazy in the least!"

Another woman informed us that she was the "top lady of the United States, and you should bow down to me." She was convinced we had poisoned her food, so she refused to eat at supper time. A 15-year-old girl, strapped down and screaming at the top of her lungs, was put directly into a seclusion room. 16-year-old Nancy was very stubborn and wouldn't let us give her a shower. What a pity that teenagers (or anyone, for that matter) are in a place like this.

We admitted meek and gentle 75-year-old Emily who had been neglected by her family. She's just getting senile. I felt sorry for her; she looked so pitiful, forlorn and lonely. We were told that her family didn't want to be bothered with caring for her anymore so she ended up in this depressing place. I'd be depressed too if my family didn't want me and put me in a place like this. It's so tragic to think there isn't a better place for such people when their family can't cope with them in society any longer. So they end up in a cold, indifferent state hospital. I hope someone can soon come up with a better idea than this.

I asked the supervisor at the charting desk, "What causes them to be this way and what could possibly be done to prevent it?"

She did not have an answer, just shrugged her shoulders and went on with her charting. I had to wonder how much the staff really care about the patients and what brought them to this place.

Thus my work was varied and interesting. It was not always physically tiring, but sometimes was very emotionally draining. After a while, it got on my nerves and I needed an outlet. I would often take my frustration out on the piano in the nurses' residence or invite a group of girls to sing with me as I played. We could make some joyful music together.

October 1, 1952: *Tonight I read the book assignment The Snake Pit, which is another novel about the appalling conditions for patients in a mental hospital. Sounds familiar?*

A female patient told me my fortune from the palm of my hand this evening. She rubbed my hand and told me that I very much wanted to get married but my mother wouldn't let me till I'm out of school. She didn't know what true words she spoke. There's nothing I would like more than to get married right now.

October 2, 1952: *Again I take up my pen and jot down the happenings of this day. We are getting in the groove more or less by now, and we know more what is expected of us. Today was a fairly routine day. There were several fights in the day room when Sophie threw a chair at Velma, Ernestine hit Melanie over the head with a metal dinner plate and they ended up in a violent tussle. Melanie bit one of the female attendants when she tried to separate her from Ernestine.*

My friend Binny is a student nurse from Jewish Hospital and is so assertive. She loves to order me around until I can feel my feathers being ruffled and rubbed the wrong way. She talked me into doing something we weren't supposed to do – release a patient from seclusion by ourselves without an attendant present. Fortunately, nothing bad happened. The supervisor lectured us severely. We probably busted our efficiency reports by doing that. Most of the time we enjoy working together. I ask God to help me to keep sweet and not be defensive. All three of the girls in my group are heavy smokers and have such different interests than I do. It's strange to be the only one to take a stand and try to stick to my principles.

October 5, 1952: *We were on duty today but didn't do anything that would classify as work since it was Sunday. We would have taken some patients to a church service on the campus but no one was well enough to go out of the building, so we brought the record player down from 4th floor and listened to hymns.*

Betty sulked in the corner all afternoon during visiting hours. We didn't know what impulsive actions she might do, so we watched her carefully. Visiting hours are hard on the patients like Betty if they don't get visitors. The atmosphere is much more cheerful when visitors come. But for those who don't get visitors, it can be depressing.

October 6, 1952: *I feel refreshed at the end of this day, and I'm enjoying life to the fullest. As I sat at the piano tonight I was thrilled when several of my colleagues gathered around me to sing the hymns I was playing.*

Today several of us worked on the men's ward on 2nd floor in N3 building. Most of them like nurses and will do most anything for us. Vernon and Max are quite the pests, though, hanging around trying to get our attention. I find I would rather work with men than women. They don't require as much painstaking persuasion as women do.

I have made a jewel of a friendship with Sophie, a student nurse from the Lankanau Hospital. We have so much in common that we can talk without any difficulty. I like her pleasant German accent. Two years ago, she came from Austria to study nursing here. She had studied in medical school four years over there, but her credits weren't accepted here.

She and I have a lot in common because we both love classical music, nature, and many other things. She's traveled extensively and teaches me a lot about Europe. I love learning to know new people who have had so many different experiences. It broadens friendships, opens up great vistas of cultural advantages and personal development for me.

October 7, 1952: *Sometimes I feel so useless here compared to how busy we were at LGH. We play games with patients, watch the ball games on television, and supervise the patients at meals and in their daily routine. But that's all part of the mental therapy, I guess. I don't know that I would want to do it all the time. What a contrast to rushing my legs off doing general duty on a surgical floor. I think I'd rather do that, though, than the slow pace we have here. Some days creep along so slowly, especially if I'm anticipating some fun activity after I get off duty.*

October 8, 1952: *At this quiet hour, I will write again about my day. On 2nd floor today there was the usual hum of activity. ECT first thing in the morning; Max insisted I play pinochle with him; Vernon is such a poor soul the way he tags around after me, begs me to give him a kiss, talks constantly about loving me and asks if I still love him. It is starting to bug me big time!*

14-year-old Johnny is here because he has epilepsy. After he told me his story, I felt so sorry for him. His father is dead and his mother is allegedly a patient here in Byberry. He has been in foster care since birth and has never seen his mother so he doesn't know if she's here or not. He says he's never been to school so cannot read or write. He likes to work and often asks if he can do something to help me. My heart goes out to him very much.

All of the patients needed love, even the violent ones. I was just one person, but I could make a smidgen of difference in someone's life with an attitude of care and concern. It was sobering to realize that I was so limited in what I could do for them.

Each day passed into nothingness except for memories. At the end of a day I couldn't say I really accomplished anything at all. The results of the nursing care we gave there were not immediately visible. Mental healing in that setting was a long-term process if it happened at all. Some will probably be there their whole life.

October 9, 1952: *This morning was almost entirely devoted to playing Chinese checkers with Larry, Joe, and Bob. Max still keeps reminding me that he's going to buy me a yellow Cadillac. Vernon* *never fails to ask if I still love him. Howard was real foxy and bothered everybody today so he was put in seclusion.*

October 13, 1952: Binny and I worked with the women on 4th floor today. These women are not as sick as the ones on 3rd floor; instead they are pleasant and friendly, but several are severely depressed. We also assisted with the daily ECT on twelve women.

Off-duty fun activities with friends

My room was often a cheerful one in the evenings when my friends gathered there. We chattered and laughed about our activities of the day, polished shoes, ate snacks, put hair in curlers, and wrote letters. I loved having them in my room. After gabbing with the gals, I was ready to crawl into my comfy bed.

Sophie and I sometimes talked until after midnight. She almost persuaded me to go with her to Europe after graduation! I would love to tour the European countries, especially with Sophie. Her family came to America from Austria when she was a little girl, and she returned to attend medical school there. Then she decided to study nursing here in America. She very much wanted to go back and see her homeland again.

One Friday night I went to Sophie's home with her. Her mother and brother were quite shy but friendly; they were still new at the English language. When they found I was just a common person too, they opened up more freely. We listened to wonderful music, and they served delicious refreshments.

Another time Allie and I cooked up this wild and brainy idea that just for fun we wanted to go sightseeing in New York City the second weekend in December; but we never did follow through on that idea.

Weekends off

It was not all work – there was some free time. I was always glad when 3:30 came on Friday, and I could go off duty for the weekend and spend time with good friends who lived and studied in the city. I took three forms of transportation – bus, elevated train, and trolley – out to 69th St. Station where Anna and Rachel met me. The three of us usually planned to do something fun together.

Sometimes we went to visit Jody and Jack who had been in my class at college, and now Jack is here in medical school. We had lovely visits in their cute apartment exchanging news, looking at pictures, and playing the pump organ. Later we visited Don who lived three blocks away. Several other friends from college often joined in the fun activities when their schedules allowed. Some weekends we planned fun activities together such as operas, concerts, and Sundays in the Park; that relieved the pressures of our work and studies.

Several of my former college friends were going to medical school in Philly. One Saturday night we all went roller skating together and took turns falling down at least once, except Bud and Bob. They were the best! Even Jerry went skating with us. He was just learning so, he fell down the most. Thankfully no one broke a bone. I don't know how many times I fell down. Next day I was terribly stiff – couldn't move without it hurting – could hardly take my uniform off by myself.

One Sunday, several of us experienced Father Divine's Heaven. It was a very unusual experience that elicited eerie feelings among our group. Afterwards, we grabbed a snack at a Horn and Hardart's Automat close by and we had a lively discussion about the strange belief system that this man Father Divine thinks he is God. There's a description of this "Father Divine's Heaven" on the internet.

Hydrotherapy

October 15, 1952: *I'm assigned to work in Hydrotherapy this week. Mrs. Roddy, the head nurse, is not very gentle with the patients. Six bathtubs are lined up in a great big room. Several of us work together to tightly wrap six patients in wet sheet packs (they end up looking like mummies), and then we lower them up to their necks in regular size bathtubs of warm water for at least an hour. This is designed to help the more violent patients calm down. Some patients end up screaming their lungs out anyway, and others almost fall asleep.*

You should have heard four of the patients yell and scream – Lollie, Lessie, Marie, and Lucy. Marie thought we were going to kill her, so she kept yelling "Murder!" at the top of her lungs. Lucy was all wound up singing "Hail, hail, the gang's all here, what the hell do we care!" It got worse before they finally decided to let the warm water quiet them down. In general, hydrotherapy is very boring. There's nothing to do from 8-11 while patients are in their packs. I'm glad I'm only assigned there for five days.

Initiation to Female Infirmary

November 3, 1952: *This was our initiation to Female Infirmary. What a depressing place it is. The patients there are quite hopeless. It literally stinks. I thought I'd keel over from the stench of urine and feces.*

Anna continually rubs the side of her head as she walks up and down the hall repeatedly mumbling, "My brain is rotting," to whoever will listen. She has been doing this so long the hair on that side of her head is rubbed off.

During the noon meal, Doris threw a baked potato at Dr. Hood, the psychiatrist, and hit her square in the head.

Binny and I worked together to shower and shampoo each one.

November 4, 1952, National Election Day: *A palpable wave of excitement permeated the air. Everyone was quite keyed up. Eisenhower was ahead so far. I hoped he would be elected. (He was.)*

Just as we were ready to crawl into bed about 10:15 last night, the fire siren blew like mad. We looked out the window and saw flames light up the sky over near the Female Infirmary. So we all quickly jerked on some clothes and dashed over there to see if they needed help. It turned out the laundry building next to the infirmary was on fire. It didn't burn down completely – only first floor was burned out – our uniforms on second floor were saved, thankfully.

November 9, 1952: *I could scream just now! I'm very depressed, having worked all weekend. Today the many visitors got on my nerves – in fact, everything got on my nerves. I'm so glad to be done with Female Infirmary. It is way too depressing.*

November 10, 1952: *This was our first day in a two-week stretch in Ergotherapy, better known in some places as Occupational Therapy. Ergo is the Latin word for "work," so it's like therapy for those who have some capability of following through on projects that staff gives them. Ergotherapy is different from other ways we work with patients. It involves the patients in directed activities: art, recreation, music, work projects, writing. This is designed to help them build their self-esteem, develop good work habits, and express themselves in useful, creative ways. The goal is to work toward the highest level of independence possible given the limitations the patient has to deal with.*

Miss S. introduced my group to our assigned patients. I am assigned to work with a 62-year-old man named Frank who has an interesting life history. I spent two hours this morning in conference with Frank and then read through his chart this afternoon.

His history: He has been in and out of Byberry over the last 40 years after he fell out of a trolley car while he was a sophomore at the university. He suffered severe brain damage from which he has never fully recovered. He was an accomplished pianist before his injury, so I hope he can learn to do that again.

After Frank and I were introduced, he repeated over and over to me, "I'm 47 years old and my name is Joseph Custard. You remind me of my mother, quiet and kind."

He goes through outlandish but rather comical maneuvers in the middle of the room as if he's performing for his mother. Says he's pretending to be in a saloon drinking whisky. He likes to clown around and tries to make me laugh. I can't help but like him and his funny little antics.

November 13, 1952: *Frank was a bit more responsive today. He and I went bowling, played checkers, and ping pong. He still talks to himself in a very preoccupied way and goes through all his silly meaningless motions. He made an attempt to play the piano and likes to dance. I have to laugh at his antics, but at the same time he can be aggravating.*

Our whole group took a field trip to one of the private mental hospitals in the area this afternoon. What luxury they have there...plush carpets on all the floors and beautiful furnishings. It's like a dazzling hotel. A person wouldn't know she/he was in a mental hospital there. The staff ratio is 2-1. I wonder what it would be like to work in that place. Such a contrast to Byberry!

November 14, 1952: *Frank and I played ping pong doubles with Rosy and Joe. Frank did pretty well. Then he played the piano until we went for a walk about 10:30. He can play chords on the piano but would have to practice a lot to get back his ability after 30 years away from it. He also said he used to play the violin, so Tony said he'll try to get him a violin from the music therapist next week. I hope he isn't leading Frank down a blind alley on that one.*

I was able to persuade Frank to go up to the blackboard and write a story for me. He wrote a short story that looked promising about his cat named Tiger. When I come back after two days off, I hope to see that he's made some progress.

November 16, 1952: *Sunday evening: I spent a wonderfully relaxing weekend at home with Mollie's family. I dreaded the trip coming back to Byberry alone after dark, but some of the Byberry nurses got on the bus at the same station. It was pitch dark from the bus to our residence, so I was very glad I had someone to walk with me the quarter mile. So now I'm back to Earth again – BANG!*

November 19, 1952: *I really don't want to leave Ergotherapy next week because Frank made some good progress today. He went up to the blackboard again and was able to write another story. I found out he can type a little bit, too. He's such a cutie...still goes through all his queer little motions.*

November 20, 1952: *It has rained nearly all day today, which makes it really nasty walking outside from building to building. There's nothing but gloom all around this place – no bright colors to look at around here – only these dull, gray buildings inside as well as outside. If I think too much about it I, can get very depressed.*

Staff conference this morning was with my case study, Mary S. For some reason she was quite upset, so we didn't accomplish much with her.

Miss B. measured all of us for our white graduate uniforms today. Everyone's uniform was to be the same distance from the bottom of the hem to the floor – 11 inches. What a thrill that was to think the last time we were measured was two years ago for our student blues. Hard to believe we are this far along already.

November 21, 1952: *This morning it was still raining all day off and on, which didn't help our spirits any. But then we can have sunshine in our hearts!*

The patients really kept us stepping lively at their weekly dance today. I was nearly exhausted by the time we were finished. Frank was so cute to dance with. He does this jig-like step without paying any attention to what his partner is doing.

These weeks are going by so fast. Today was our last day in Ergo. Frank wanted to kiss me goodbye. I'm really going to miss him. I finished my case study, so that's off my chest now.

Initiation to the Women's Ward

November 24, 1952: *Four of us were initiated to the women's 2nd East Floor in N-6, which was quite a dramatic experience – another smelly place! We gave bed baths, cleaned up after incontinent patients, treated bedsores, and listened to the constant yapping. Mildred keeps saying to herself, "That's my baby!" Iyana gives forth constantly with, "Tttttttttttttt...tttt". Patients have deteriorated to the point of being completely hopeless, it seems. Even Female Infirmary was never like* *this. But staff tells us we will learn to like it and will hate to leave. Sure! I'll believe it when I see it.*

Dr. E. assigned us to observe three manic-depressive patients. Their attention span was very short, and their moods were so changeable. I learned a lot there, but I know I am still very naïve when it comes to understanding the behavior of mentally ill patients.

November 27, 1952: *Happy Thanksgiving! I can imagine this was a happy day for many people. As for me, it was spent working 2nd E as usual. The odor was so bad we were thankful we were only working there. There's really no way to do productive therapy of any kind with them. All we did was give baths and change wet beds for the 30 patients. We changed bed linens only twice today. I never changed so many bed linens with urine and feces in all my life, and I hope I never will again.*

During the noisy hubbub, Joyce and I tried to get Mabel to cooperate at mealtime and she became very agitated. She screamed at us:

"Leave me alone! I hate those darned nurses' caps you wear. They look like inverted teapots. Those black bands on them are contraceptive bands so you don't get pregnant!"

She referred to the black velvet bands on our caps that designate those of us from LGH as senior nursing students. By this time, we knew we could expect anything to come out of a patient's mouth so we don't take it personally.

December 1, 1952: *Winnie and I were assigned these two weeks to the Women's 4th floor in N3. This is where the Occupational Therapy (O.T) department has more advanced craft classes for the patients. How refreshing it is to work a full day in O.T. without any other classes.*

Mrs. L., the therapist, is so sweet and everyone likes her a lot. The women there are not as sick and so we could converse with them more easily. They loved painting Christmas decorations. It helps to cheer up the whole place. Winnie and I are both teaching our patients to crochet doilies. The whole group joined in singing around the piano while I played familiar songs.

December 11, 1952: *I started the day on 2nd East long enough to give Mamie her bath and change her bed linens. She called me every dirty name she could think of. That experience might have set the tone for the entire day but, when I considered the source, I felt great compassion for her and could let it slide off and out of my mind.*

Later I went back to the O.T. department and helped Betty make a little mattress and pillow for the doll bed she was working on.

December 12, 1952: *This was our last day in O.T. and we hated to leave it. Mrs. L. was generous and gave me an "A" in my efficiency report. After dinner I went back over to 2nd East and had fun helping two patients paint Christmas pictures on the windows. I also helped decorate the ward for the Christmas party this afternoon.*

At the end of this day, I feel quite empty. The psychology test was really difficult. I don't think I made a very good grade, but I just hope at least I passed it. Wanda and I had studied awhile this morning, but we didn't learn much by cramming at the last minute.

Such a crazy time as we had singing hymns on the way to take the test – "I Need Thee Every Hour," "All Things Are Possible," "Faith of Our Fathers," etc. We needed to boost our spirits in any way we could.

Initiation to 2nd West

December 15, 1952: *This was the first of seven days with the women in 2nd West, and what a place! We were shocked to the very soles of our feet. More horrible smells and gruesome sight – nude patients crouched in the hallways and dayroom, feces and urine most any place you look, women menstruating without sanitary pads. Where are the attendants? Who is it they are trying to rehabilitate here, anyway?*

December 16, 1952: Happy Birthday to me! *I am 22 years old today and already I feel like an old woman. I certainly celebrated this* *day in royal style and fashion. It was shower day on 2nd West. The patients are incapable of cleaning themselves well enough, so I had to get into the shower one at a time with them. Consequently I was showered almost as much as my patients were. That is such a hectic procedure. Also, I trimmed their toenails. They hollered if I tickled their feet. What a way to celebrate a birthday. Ugh!*

December 17, 1952: *It was my turn to give morning medicines today. Thorazine was one of the drugs that we gave to violent and catatonic patients.*

By the time we had our coffee hour and took patients for a walk, it was lunchtime. Such a raucous time we have at meals. The grabbers are so messy – they gobble their food down and then grab someone else's before we can stop them. If anyone could hear us yell at them, they would be shocked.

[Author's note about medication: condensed from People and Discoveries: Science Odyssey – "Drug for treating schizophrenia identified 1952." One of the first psychotropic drugs to be developed was Thorazine. It eventually became the drug of choice for schizophrenia. It had a calming effect on violent patients without sedating them too much, allowing them to live a nearly normal life. The drug was introduced first to state hospitals. They began testing the drug at institutions where the most hopeless cases were housed, including Byberry. The results were convincing, even miraculous, with some patients. Catatonic patients who had stood in one spot without moving for weeks and violent patients who had to be restrained could now interact with others and be unsupervised at times.

Side effects and drawbacks to the drug were revealed early on. For example, one side effect of the drug was a severe tremor resembling Parkinson's disease. Some patients also developed what was called the "Thorazine shuffle" when they walked (http://www.pbs.org/wgbh/aso/databank/entries/dh52dr.html).

December 19, 1952: *It was shower day again and believe me, it was shower! Wanda and I wore bandannas when we washed the patients, but it didn't do one speck of good; our hair got wet and straight as a* *stick anyway. Then we helped monitor the women during dinner to make sure they didn't throw their food at each other.*

The patients watched a real cute movie, "Snow White and the Seven Dwarfs," after the meal. Binny and I painted Christmasy stuff on the windows most of the afternoon and helped trim the tree until we went off duty at 3:30.

Leaving Byberry

December 19, 1952: *Such mingled feelings I have tonight as I sit down and write for the last time here at Byberry. It's been like a sisterhood. When I think of leaving the place, all the friends I've made, and the nurses I've worked with for three months, I could cry. The group pictures came today and I asked for autographs as a way to remember each of my friends. It is a dismal feeling to be torn apart and go in different directions. Such grand friendships we have known here. I dread for it to come to an end – and yet I want tomorrow to come so I can go home. I must get busy with the rest of my packing.*

December 20, 1952: *Bye, bye Byberry! As we were parting, it was painful to think that we are leaving forever and ever. It brought sadness to our hearts. Maybe I'll be back again as a graduate sometime. A small part of me thinks I would like to work here after I graduate. It's been a fascinating learning experience, although it isn't a happy place. Instead, it was a wild and wooly three months' challenge to treat the patients as human beings instead of like caged animals. Now I am going back to the sheltering arms of LGH.*

[Author's note: There are many historical information and pictures about Byberry on the Internet. Search www.philadephiastatehospital.com for "The story of Byberry 1906-2006".]

During World War II, many Mennonite men who were conscientious objectors for religious convictions had refused to go to war, but were instead willing to do alternate service and be assigned to work in places few outsiders got to see or wanted to work in — mental institutions like Philadelphia State Hospital.

In May1946 after World War II, *LIFE* magazine published a scathing photographic exposé about the horrendous warehouse conditions in which patients lived at Byberry. It was broadcast on National Public Radio in 2009. More information is available at: http://www.pbs.org/wgbh/americanexperience/features/primary-resources/lobotomist-bedlam-1946/.

After their experiences in mental hospitals were over, those from Byberry and other such institutions were so moved to start a national association called Mennonite Mental Health that helped educate professional workers at state hospitals. Dedicated people worked to improve the lives of the vulnerable people who lived in those state institutions.This church-related group then organized and established several private, church-sponsored mental hospitals that provide compassionate care to those who struggle with mental illnesses and disabilities. Those hospitals are still in existence today.

Since this societal cancer was exposed to the public, mentally ill patients now receive more humane treatment. Extensive research on psychotropic medications has resulted in fewer patients needing to be hospitalized for long periods of time. Many psychiatric patients have been discharged from state hospitals and are maintained with medications on an out-patient status.

Chapter 22
Return to LGH

Enjoying Christmas Season

December 21, 1952: *It's so good to be back on familiar home territory again. Monday I got up bright and early to begin work on 3rd East. It was a rather strenuous day because Joyce and I had to get used to being bedside nurses again. It is such a different kind of nursing from Byberry where we regularly sat around and played games with the patients.*

This evening I joined the other gals as we watched Dickens' "A Christmas Carol" on TV. We chatted and giggled around the decorated tree in the living room for a long time as the blinking lights signaled that it was Christmas Eve. It was 1:15 a.m. before we decided to go to bed.

December 25, 1952: MERRY CHRISTMAS!! *I worked a day shift, and it hasn't seemed at all like Christmas Day by any stretch of the imagination. If it wasn't for the Christmas music on the TVs and radios in the patients' rooms, I would have never known it was Christmas. But be that as it may, everyone had the "Spirit of Idleness" today. Several of us went caroling through the hospital with Mrs. K. Life has taken on a more or less settled routine now that we are back at good old LGH.*

December 31, 1952, 11:30 p.m.: *The last day of 1952! What will this next year bring? It snowed furiously all afternoon. Again we went round and round in busy circles on duty. It was Sallie's last day of work so we had a little going away party for her – we will miss her a lot.*

At 3:30 I dashed off the unit, got my stuff together, and caught the 4:15 bus home. I didn't even take time to change out of uniform. Due to the snow, everything turned white and slippery real fast and the bus was 20 minutes late getting into town. Carl met me at the bus terminal and we enjoyed a good supper as always at his mother's table before we went to an inspirational Watch Night service at church. Now we are back at his home safely, snug and warm while it is terrifically stormy outside. Roads are very treacherous.

January 10, 1953 A letter to Carl: *Your welcomed letter arrived earlier today. New Year's greetings from the drippy, soggy, slushy city of Lancaster. Isn't this the awfulest weather? It certainly is not fun slopping through the puddles with freshly polished white shoes. What a mess to have to jump puddles.*

We have been so frightfully busy. When we do get off duty exhausted, all we can do is flop on our beds and sleep. So I apologize if it seems as though my thoughts have not wandered in your direction lately. Sometimes work takes priority, eh?

As a senior, I took my turn to be second in charge of the unit tonight. This is so we learn how to manage the unit, delegate tasks, and see that everything is done properly and runs smoothly. It carries a lot of added responsibilities, e.g. order needed supplies, admit/assess new patients, make rounds with doctors and transfer their orders to the Kardex, order medications, delegate tasks to other staff, and do lots of charting/paperwork.

Within one hour we admitted five new patients and had to prepare one of them for the O.R right away. Thankfully there was enough staff that I could delegate different duties. I flew around the unit with so much stuff on my mind and so much pressure to do things in a timely manner. Well, so much for that rigamarole. I'll write more another time. Love, M.

January 14, 1953 An emotionally charged letter to Carl about my frustrations: *"Here I am again, giving you the low-down from LGH. Thanks for your letter today. It cheered me up! I was in a very disturbed state of mind, and rather depressed. I still am, though not as much as I was before your letter came. I probably shouldn't write to you when my nervous system has been taxed to the limit. I need a new supply of patience. What does the Bible say about "tribulation gives patience"? I've had plenty of tribulation but no patience today. At least not yet.*

The root of all this complaining is the fact that we have a new supervisor on 3rd East who sits around and does crossword puzzles while we are working ourselves to death. Imagine this:

"Miss Minter, will you please make rounds with Dr. Welch?"

"Miss Minter, please copy these orders."

"Miss Minter, take this report to the office."

Grrrrrrr – rrrr! Sounds like she is trying to delegate tasks but every one of those tasks are her responsibility, not mine. The unit is in a constant state of confusion and chaos, in my opinion. No one knows what they are doing because there is no organization. And that, to me, is the most essential thing in running a busy, booming unit.

Tuesday the place was a riot. I was on evening duty and we were so busy giving intensive care to six fresh cataract post-ops. A cataract patient requires lots of care because the person has to lie flat on her/his back with sandbags on both sides of the head for several days. This is to immobilize the head and prevent movement that might slow the healing of the surgical site. Since they can't move, we also have to spoon feed them.

All the T & As (tonsillectomies and adenoidectomies) are observed constantly for signs of hemorrhage and spitting up blood all over the place. One patient went into shock for us and we scurried around lowering his head in the Trendelenburg position (propping up the foot of the bed so his head was lower than his feet) and other measures to restore his equilibrium.

Wednesday was chopped up, meaning I worked like a horse till 12:30 then Miss F. comes around asking if I'd leave and come back to work charge nurse on the evening shifts the rest of the week. The regular evening charge nurse had called and said that she wasn't coming to work anymore. I don't blame her. She was probably turned off by all the chaos in the place.

By that time I was so fed up with the place and the people I felt like quitting myself. But since I'm a student I can't just call in and say I'm not coming to work anymore. Well, I guess I could but what would that solve? So I dutifully went off duty. After taking some deep breaths and a nap my fuming heart simmered down. At 7 p.m. I went back to work and things naturally went better with me in charge!

Maybe I'm a soft touch or something, but I am a senior student who wants to do what is in the best interests of the patients in my care. If that means being inconvenienced occasionally, then so be it. Only seniors are allowed to be in charge on evening duty, so I got the job since it's quite a specialized group of patients – cataract removals, tonsillectomies, etc.

Another irritant is the nurse's aide. Now, I don't mind working hard but the least they could do is give me an aide who doesn't have to be told every little thing to do and then I have to supervise the job on top of that yet. I'd rather do it all myself, but with all my other work to do that's not feasible, either.

So now, except for Friday night, I'm scheduled to be on evening duty for the rest of the week. At least I have off Friday night. Maybe we can arrange a date. So much for the thrills and joys of being a senior.

Having said all that, I'll shut up, quiet down, and relax. This is one of those times that I get so fed up with the place that it would be easy to just quit. But I'm too close to the end to let that happen. Oh, well, only 7 ½ months yet to go and then I can flap my wings and take off.

Sunday evening went fairly easy compared to the previous ones. Only one thing irked me: a patient requested a pain medication an hour before his bedtime. At the time I was in the process of doing a dressing change so I assured him I'd give him his pain medicine at bedtime. But 1/2 hour later his son came stomping in to the nurses' station and said in a demanding voice:

"Can my father have something for pain, or must I call a doctor?"

To prevent any further upset feelings I said: "Sure, I'll give him something now."

I quickly finished the dressing and got the man's medication. A half hour later, one of his doctors called asking why his patient isn't getting his medication. Fifteen minutes later his other doctor called. I reassured both of them that I had already given him pain medication. The doctors were perturbed that they had been bothered. Can't say as I blame them.

I reported to the patient that both of his doctors had called and that satisfied him. There was something amusing about the incident after it was all over. I call it the "power of one to get something done". Hey, that rhymes.

Gotta sign off for now. This letter is so long, you're probably sound asleep already. My love always, M"

January 25, 1953: *Thank goodness, tomorrow is my last day on 3rd East! I hope I never see that place again as long as I live. The nurse in charge and I were the only ones on duty, so you know who did the work? Me! Then she had the guts to ask me what she should do. A supervisor! She doesn't do a blessed thing but sit around – doesn't even make rounds with the doctors. Today we caught her taking spiritus frumenti from the medicine cabinet! (it's an alcoholic drink that is occasionally ordered as a medication)*

Chapter 23
Emergency Room Rotation

For the next three weeks, the "Receiving Ward," or emergency room (E.R.) as it is called most places, turned out to be a whole different kind of nursing. Mrs. S. was easy to work with as well as the nurses' aide. The orderlies were okay too, but they liked to hang out at the nurses' station and tell off-color jokes.

January 26, 1953: I just love the work there. There is a lot to learn and remember. Heavy responsibility lies in our hands. We get everything from smashed fingers, ruptured appendix, common colds, shotgun wounds, to broken vertebrae. It calls out the very best in us to remain poised and calm in the face of an emergency.

Three times today I went out with the ambulance and was so absorbed that I forgot I had a class from 1-2 pm. Thankfully it was only the Army Nurse telling about the opportunities if we join the Army nurse Corps, and she didn't take roll call.

Seniors have interviews with Mrs. K this week. She wants us to present an outline of what we hope to do after we are finished with the program in September. I'm undecided yet about whether I'll look for a job back home near my parents or plan to work here for a while. In professional procedures class, Mrs. K. gave us helpful suggestions on applying for jobs.

January 30, 1953: *The last ambulance run this evening took us to an old rickety house. We had to walk on a narrow wooded trail back through the trees before arriving at the run-down house. A foul odor emanated from the whole place. Inside the house, the atmosphere was even worse that we had imagined – simply revolting. Three small rooms littered with junk and thick with dirt. I can't adequately describe the putrefying atmosphere!*

There, in the far corner on the floor, wrapped in a dirty blanket on a rusty bedspring, lay a shriveled up elderly woman curled into a ball moaning with severe abdominal pain. Her middle-aged son was pacing the floor, helplessly wringing his hands and crying:

"She got sick two days ago and I didn't know what to do," he told us. A next door neighbor had called for the ambulance.

We managed to lift her on to the litter and carry her out through all the trash and the trees to the ambulance. It's beyond me how some people can live like that. She ended up being admitted to the hospital and having abdominal surgery, so I never saw her again.

I'm on call tonight and the ambulance driver just now paged me, so I have to be prepared for anything when I get there. Meeting an emergency makes my heart race faster, but it is all about staying calm and alert.

One disadvantage of working in the E.R. was that the patients were either discharged home, to another facility, or transferred to a hospital room. It was next to impossible to follow up to know whether they got well or died.

Some nights there were no ambulance calls, but we were kept fairly busy with walk-ins that were less critical cases e.g. sprained ankle, bruised arm, pneumonia, appendectomy, etc.

I couldn't decide if I liked it there after all. My impression on several nights was one of utter repulsion. When there was not enough work to keep the ambulance driver and orderlies busy, the nursing station turned out to be the general loafing center. Such filthy talk as I heard from those guys. It was sickening. That place had a bad reputation for that, especially on evening duty. When I politely asked them not to talk like that my request was totally ignored. I just prayed to God that I would be able to forget all that nasty stuff.

February 3, 1953: *A real bad accident case was admitted -- a man injured by a "hit and run" driver. He was a dirty, bloody mess from head to foot plus several fractures, so we sent him to surgery immediately.*

We admitted a squalling child who had fallen to the pavement when his dad tripped and fell while carrying him. The dad wasn't hurt but the child could sure raise the roof with his howling. When we took the child up for a skull X-ray, the technician showed me how to run the machine while she held the child down. That was a big job in itself. So now I know how to run the X-ray machine. How about that? Fortunately the child didn't have a fractured skull.

An 18-month-old child was brought in with a 2nd degree burn of the finger after he stuck it into a hot potato. He had a lusty cry, too.

Jack, George, and I went to Lititz via ambulance for a patient with an acute case of kidney stones. He was in terrific pain that responded immediately to an injection of pain medication. That's a sampling of our evening.

This Friday night I'm scheduled to be in charge there all by myself. That's the night when lots of emergency stuff happens. Won't that be just ducky? Watch me get somebody who was stabbed, shot, or run over. Well, that's what makes for variety. I like to be able to fix these people up and hope they get better. That's the satisfaction of being a nurse. My time in emergency room will be over the end of this week. I'm rather sad to have it end so soon.

Chapter 24
The Final Countdown to Graduation

Different schedules and shifts

After finishing my rotation in the emergency room, I returned to routine bedside nursing and worked wherever and whenever the supervisors decided to send me. It was quite a variety of shifts and types of patients. This would be routine from now until the end of my student days in September because I had been through all the rotations.

February 15, 1953: *I was asked to fill in a very busy day shift on 1st floor Maternity. It was just Jackie and me with 23 patients. I don't like to be so rushed like that. We can't do the patients justice that way. Tomorrow I start on 3rd West in the new part of the hospital. That will be a nice change.*

February 17, 1953: *I'm finding out 3rd West isn't too bad. It's like all medical floors – stacks of medications, fussy cardiac patients, lots of full bed baths, and back rubs to give. I'll be there one week on day duty and four weeks of night duty. I'll be glad to get on nights again for a change. Miss C. is the supervisor and she's very organized. What a blessing.*

I had my wisdom teeth X-rayed again today at Dr. Unser's office, and he said I must have all four of my wisdom teeth extracted as they are coming in crooked and crowding my other teeth. Now I'll have to be thinking about that scenario. Not a happy thought. I hate going to dentists! At least this time the hospital will pay the bill.

February 19, 1953: *I don't know what's wrong with me tonight – I feel half-way depressed, and then again I just lack ambition. It is that odd sensation of wanting something but not quite knowing what I want. I hope I'll pull out of it soon.*

Yesterday I had 5 full bed baths to give, so I took my time and was able to get everything done in good time.

Mrs. Morris is a dear white-haired lady who loves to knit and crochet pretty things. She and I have lots to talk about when I'm giving her a bath or backrub.

Old Pappy Sayers is a comical soul who is so absent-minded. He has trouble finding things like his glasses, hearing aid, and false teeth. They are usually somewhere close by, even in his bed linens sometimes. We have to carefully search the linens so that we don't inadvertently send personal items to the laundry.

Mr. Eller calls for help when he has to go to the bathroom several times a night. Even though it's a nuisance getting him to and from the bathroom, it's better than having him soil the bed or fall and break a leg.

Instead of ringing her bell, Mrs. Hart pounds on her bedpan when she wants attention and wakes the other patients up. Such a racket that makes at 2 a.m.!

A letter from my family says they have the weeks counted till they will be coming for my graduation in May. I can hardly wait. My heart skips a couple beats every time I think of it.

I wrote a letter to Carl last week but forgot to mail it. When I came back to my room it was gone. Everyone I asked knew nothing about it. I do hope someone mailed it. Maybe the house mother censored it, for all I know. Maybe she took my $7 that is missing, too. Strange things are happening around here.

It's 1:30 a.m. and I'm writing this journal in bits and pieces while on night duty. I'm about to fall asleep because I had so little sleep today, so guess I'd better walk around awhile and check on my patients.

One evening, Diana told me Mrs. K wanted to see me right away. Oh dear! What dreadful thing had I done now? Come to find out she had gotten several calls from my parents trying to let me know that my Uncle Fred died this week and they wanted me to come home for the funeral. Dad called again then later, and I talked to both him and mother. I felt so homesick and sad. My uncle was the last living close relative on my birth mother's side of the family.

Mrs. K. would not agree to give me the time off since it was not one of my parents or siblings who died. So the decision was already made for me. I was sorry not to be able to go for the funeral there in Oklahoma. Airfare would have been prohibitive, anyway.

Beginning to work a 44 hour week

One day in March, Mrs. K. announced that starting next week we will work only 44 hours a week instead of the 48 hour weeks we have been working. It meant we would have an extra half day off each week instead of only one. We would be permitted to have two overnights in a week. It was one of the new government labor laws. How about that? I didn't think I'd live to see it.

March 18, 1953: *A brief update: My last remaining night duty tour was nothing exciting. We've completed most of the classwork and specialty rotations. I'm not journaling very faithfully because the work on the units is routine now as we wind down toward graduation. The only breaks in the monotony have been a few of the moneyed patients who think they are not getting their money's worth of service here. It sure isn't because we're not trying to give the best care possible.*

On April 2, I began a five week stretch on 2nd West. Miss G. seemed easier to get along with this time for some reason. Thank goodness I had vacation to look forward to after that.

We seniors had only eight more weeks till graduation day. What a thrill – I could hardly wait. Then our student days would be over September 12 when our full three years ended.

April 4, 1953: *We were powerfully busy today with 6 surgeries that required lots of attention and care. I gave 8 enemas besides my other work. I didn't have to go on duty until 10 a.m., which I don't like on a day that we don't have classes. Seems like the day just drags on and on until 7 p.m. without a break. Then it's too late for any evening activity, so I'm stuck in my room for the rest of the evening.*

April 5, 1953: *Today was my day off, but I was so depressed when I got up this morning. I thought I just had to get away – clear away – where I could forget there was ever a place called LGH. I decided to spend part of my day off at the lovely city park since it was such a gorgeous, warm, and balmy day. I had an urge to be alone with God and nature and forget I ever had a care or trouble in the world, so I spent time on the beautiful fragrant wooded trail all by myself. It was a wonderful time. My spirits were boosted tremendously – at least for now.*

My wisdom teeth extraction was scheduled in the O.R. for May 2. I sent the consent form for dental surgery to the folks for them to sign. What a bummer to look forward to such a drastic procedure. It happened to be scheduled on the first day of my vacation, too. Double bummer!

Also got the word that the beautiful blonde Dr. Elsa at Byberry was hospitalized as a patient at University Hospital, Psychiatric Ward. I thought she was a good psychiatrist when I worked there. Psychiatrists are people with problems, too. It can happen to the best.

April 6, 1953: *Riley and I had a doozy of a shift on evening duty. We admitted two patients who were brought in by ambulance – one was a stat surgery for a perforated ulcer that went up to surgery at 10:55. We weren't able to start our charting till 11 and had 8 p.m. temperatures to chart also. We got off at 11:45 and still thought of a dozen things we might have left undone. When I worked night duty I did not like it when the evening nurses left stuff for me to finish, so I try not to do that to someone else.*

April 17, 1953: *This is my week of working PRN which means wherever and whenever I'm needed. Here is a good example of the crazy schedule this week: Worked 11 p.m. - 7 a.m., tried to sleep a few hours between 10 a.m. and 2 p.m., then back to work 3 - 11:30. The next day I doubled back, worked 10:30 a.m. -.7 p.m., and had trouble keeping awake. That is a brutal schedule. It's no wonder I am depressed. I believe that sleep deprivation affects my moods more than anything else.*

Deanna and I were on night duty when we changed to Daylight Saving Time, so we lost that precious hour of sleep that I can't afford to lose. Tomorrow we have several surgeries scheduled, so it will be a very busy day shift.

Ah yes, a few more days until I'm released from this drudgery for 3 whole weeks of vacation. Of course, something could happen that would prevent it so I never fully count on anything. Hardly seems possible it's almost a year since my last one. Nothing exciting ever happens at work anymore. It's just one monotonous grind sometimes.

Chapter 25
Dental Surgery and Goodbye to the Books

Putting away books

May 2, 1953: *It gave me great satisfaction to stow away my books today. We have completed all the basic foundation subjects of our program. Now they can stay put aside until time to review for state board exams. UGH – the very thought of them gives me cold shivers up and down my vertebral column.*

Undergoing dental surgery

May 15, 1953: *I have focused on wisdom teeth extraction the last two weeks so haven't done any journaling. Going under sodium pentathol anesthesia was a feathery feeling of floating. All four of my wisdom teeth were extracted, and I had 1000 cc of intravenous glucose. For 24 hours I was completely out of it because they kept me pretty well doped up with Demerol painkiller. When I came out of the fog, my jaws were so sore.*

Bless his heart, Carl brought me flowers when he visited me in the nurses' infirmary on Saturday. I was definitely not a pretty sight with my face badly swollen. He told me I looked like the little round-faced girl in the commercial for Campbell's Soup.

When I was discharged after four days, Mollie's mother came to take me home. I went straight to bed with an ice bag on my aching jaws. I couldn't open my mouth far enough to get a spoon in. Just drank cool liquids with a straw. Now my jaws are pretty well healed. I'm so glad that's over.

Chapter 26
Graduation and Vacation

My parents and siblings arrive

May 17, 1953: *This morning, Mollie's family and I were all ready for church when a blue car with Kansas license plates drove up to the house. My parents and siblings had arrived for my graduation. Two minutes later and we would have gone off to church, and missed them. We didn't go to church but instead I went with them to the cottage that Carl's folks have offered them to stay in. There we had a grand reunion. Ate breakfast together, we had worship and just enjoyed being a family again. It was so good to see them, I could hardly contain my joy and excitement.*

Other activities during the next week

Baccalaureate service was that Sunday evening after they arrived. It was exciting to get all dressed up in our white graduate uniforms and caps.

Monday, my family and I went sightseeing in Philadelphia – Independence Hall, Wanamakers, Betsy Ross House, and the Philadelphia Zoo. We ate our lunch on the zoo picnic grounds using the setup Dad had very cleverly designed for the trip. It was very unique and handy; it consisted of a small gas stove and a special suitcase fitted with pans, utensils, and staple foods. Dad's famous ingenious creativity came through loud and clear. That night we stayed in a cozy cabin near Washington, D.C.

Tuesday it rained nearly all day, just a steady pouring rain as we drove south to Washington, D.C. In spite of the rain, we toured the Capitol, Washington Monument, Lincoln Memorial, Medical Museum, Natural History Museum, Smithsonian Institute, Mt. Vernon, and Washington Cathedral.

Under clear blue skies on Wednesday, we drove on to Gettysburg and the Civil War museum, had a guided tour of the Gettysburg

Battlefield, spread our lunch on a big rock at a lovely picnic spot in a woodsy area, and thoroughly enjoyed basking in the warm sunshine.

Graduation at last (though not officially finished with student nursing yet)

May 19, 1953: *My sister washed and ironed my white uniform so nicely for me, and the family brought it with them when they came for the graduation ceremony. Before the ceremony, our entire class was decked out in our graduate caps and uniforms for a picture on the steps in front of the Fondersmith Nurses' Home. Our uniform hemlines mentioned earlier were noticeably all the same lengths, eleven inches from the floor. It's a good conversation piece!*
[This picture is prominently displayed in my living room.]

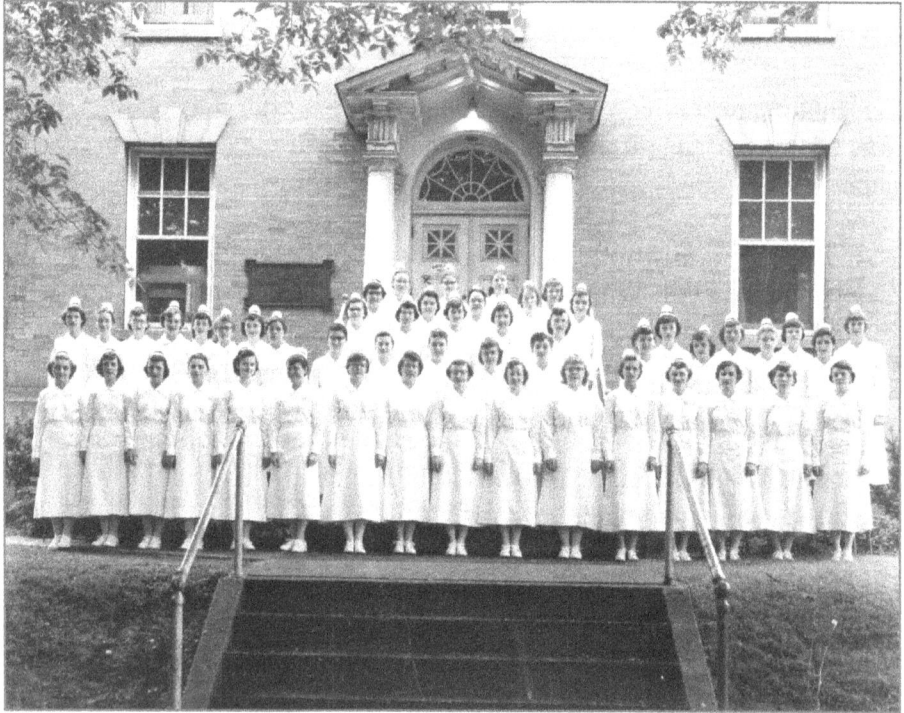

At the graduation ceremony, we received our diplomas and a gold-colored pin to wear with the name of the Lancaster General Hospital School of Nursing engraved on it. A reception afterwards at the Iris Club that night was a very lovely occasion.

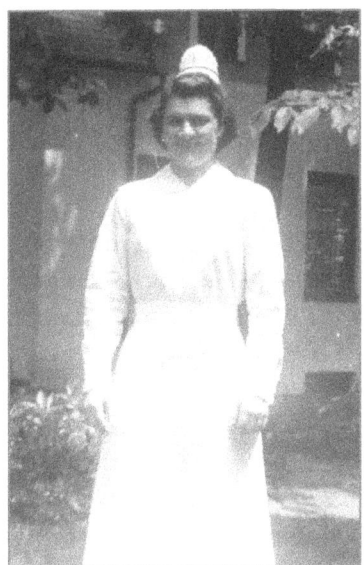 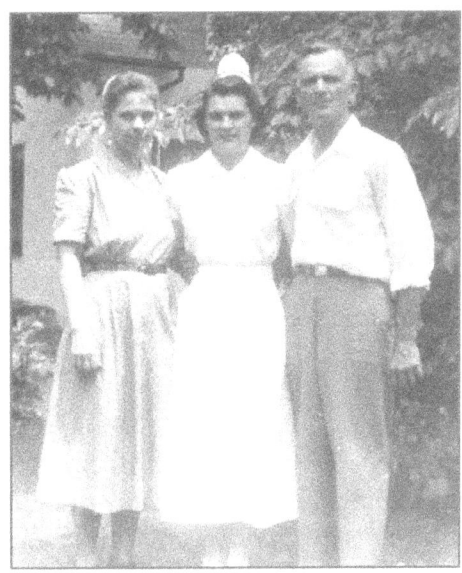

Left: Marilyn in her graduate cap and uniform.   Right: Marilyn with her parents Sam and Ruth Minter

After the ceremony and reception were over, we had to give our pins and diplomas back to Mrs. K. We were not officially finished with this place until September 10; I've often wondered why graduation was in May instead of September. We had to go back to the drudgery of work on the wards until then.

Saturday, the intermediate students honored us with a very nice buffet of snacks. Carl came and presented me with a pretty corsage of bright red carnations. All this special attention was very exciting and exhilarating.

More time with family

My vacation officially ended and I went back to work day shifts on Women's Surgical Ward, but the family stayed around for another week. Every day they picked me up after I got off work at 3 p.m. and we spent time together visiting with our good friends.

June 4, 1953: *Last Friday after my shift was over, we all enjoyed touring the Hershey Chocolate Factory and nearby Rose Gardens. The*

flowers were at their absolute peak and were so beautiful. I took my first ever ride on the huge roller coaster. Wow – that was scary. Mom was scared, too. She had to hold her false teeth in and vowed she would never get on one again. My siblings teased her a lot about having to hold her teeth in. They boldly went on several other rides.

In the evening, the family ate supper together around the big table in the cabin. We had hoped to have a picnic outside, but because it had begun to rain we had to have it inside. It didn't dampen our spirits at all.

Carl spent the evening in his room preparing the valedictorian speech he was scheduled to give at his college graduation the next day. At 10 p.m., he put up his books, came over to the cabin, and we surprised him with his graduation gifts. With the speech hanging over him, it was easy to see he wasn't relaxed.

I was feeling weepy for some reason when Dad drove me back to Lancaster. I couldn't keep from crying on his shoulder when he left me off at my dorm. My patience had become frayed at the edges because I had hoped maybe Carl would offer to drive me back since we hadn't had time together for several weeks.

Let me explain a bit: the strain at the end of the school year was affecting Carl like it did last year when he was yearbook editor. It was not quite as bad this time, but it robbed us of the closeness between us. It was hard to wait patiently until he was free from the pressure of studies, year-end exams, and two speeches.

June 5, 1953: *Well, today was the big day of Carl's college graduation! I really had a rush of events all day. I got up at 6 a.m. really tired because I hadn't gotten to sleep till 2 a.m.*

Mollie and I buzzed up to the college graduation ceremonies. Carl's speech went well. He acted so composed and confident. However, earlier he had told us he was very nervous. I had to come back to work immediately, so we didn't have any time together. What a bummer. I was in charge of the unit the rest of the evening.

Another day at the beach

On my day off, Mollie's family and my family spent a perfect day at the beach near Atlantic City, New Jersey. The sun was shining brightly and the cool, ocean breeze gently fanned our faces. We browsed the stores on the boardwalk and ate our picnic lunch sprawled out on the soft sand. My siblings enjoyed leaping into the waves and breakers. It was their first time to experience the vast ocean. We arrived home about 9:45 pm, tired, salty, sandy, and sunburned.

The next day the children begged to go horseback riding, so Mollie took them over to Everts to ride while the mothers and fathers went for a drive; this left Carl and me at home alone to thrash out some of the decisions confronting him about the post-graduation options he was struggling with. I discovered that he had difficulty making decisions.

Saying goodbye to family

Finally, after two wonderful weeks together, the day had come for my family to return to Kansas. We said our last tearful farewells, and I came back to ward duty again as they sped on their way to the church conference in Ohio.

Dad called me the next day before I went to work to tell me what happened after they left. Soon after they got on the Pennsylvania Turnpike, they discovered they had turned the wrong way. Instead of heading to Ohio they were already halfway to New York City! I could hardly believe my ears. So they decided to drive on and spend a few days in the Big Apple instead of the church conference.

After they were back home in Kansas, Dad wrote to me about their NYC adventure. When they were looking for a hotel downtown, he stopped to ask a policeman for directions.

Dad told him, "We are a missionary family of five looking for a hotel. Can you help us?"

The policeman graciously helped them find an economical hotel room and suggested things to see in New York City. What a helpful cop! They said they enjoyed their three days in the Big Apple.

I was puzzled as to why Dad would use the "missionary family" label to ask for help when he was a mid-western wheat and cattle farmer. It didn't seem like something my dad would do. After I thought about it, in one sense of the word he and mom really were missionaries. They frequently and generously donated their time and money to help individuals and many Christian missionary causes.

June 22, 1953: *For the next week, Miss B. is coaching me on how to do charge duty as a senior. She is a perfectionist and rarely goes off on time herself. She thinks no one can do things quite like she can. Once she stayed till 7 p.m.*

This coming Friday is my last day on Women's Surgical. I will not be sorry to leave that place and move on to greener pastures.

June 28, 1953: *Mollie and I are spending four days of vacation at the beach near Ocean City. We woke up at 4:30 this morning, packed a lunch, ate breakfast, and were off to get the 6:10 bus that arrived in Ocean City about 11:30 a.m. We settled in to a real nice room at the Seaview Hotel right on the beach that we had reserved earlier.*

July 2, 1953: *This whole week we practically lived in our bathing suits and shorts. It was such fun jumping the waves, laying in the sun (I had learned my lesson about laying out in the hot midday sun too long), window shopping along the boardwalk, sightseeing, and going to a couple of movies – Tonight We Sing and Desert Song. It was relaxing to sleep late, eat only two meals a day, and just goof off. It was a wonderful, refreshing vacation.*

Work on 4th Floor East

July 5, 1953: *This was my first day on 4th East, another one of the new hospital wings – I'm scheduled to work one week on days and four weeks on nights. It was hard to come back to work after such a grand vacation, but we have the inspiring thought of only eight more* *weeks to work as students. How anxious I am to know what the future holds for me. Time will tell.*

My interview with Mrs. K. went better than I thought it would. I told her that I wanted to stay at LGH until after I took my State Board Exams on October 30 and 31. She then hired me to work nights in Labor and Delivery starting in September. So far, everything was working out beautifully.

July 6, 1953: *When I went for the mail, what should I find but a card from Carl saying he has been assigned to do voluntary service in Kansas only 100 miles from my parents' home. I decided to work here at LGH until the end of October when I take State Boards and then hightail it to Kansas. In the meantime, I will explore job opportunities close to my parents' home. Carl and I have talked about getting married next summer. It's a great life...mapping the future together.*

I must finish my surgical patient case study or I'll have my overnight privilege taken away next week. That will be my last case study. Hallelujah!

July 11, 1953: *Several of the doctors are on vacation now so the whole hospital is resting quietly, taking a vacation, too. 4th East census is way down and we aren't busy at all, in fact we nearly break our necks trying to find enough to do. Ironically that is almost as tiring as working hard for eight hours. Figure that one out.*

July 12, 1953: *Today was the big day for Carl to leave for his voluntary service assignment. His family and I had a devotional time together before we took him to the train station to go to Kansas. His mom packed a lunch for him to take along. She was very tearful sending her "little boy" off halfway across the continent. The train pulled in at exactly 7:34 p.m. Carl and I said our goodbyes – oh! I could hardly let go of holding him close!*

Now I am almost ready to go to work. How will I ever keep awake all night with only a couple hours of sleep in the last two days? Maybe thinking about the many recent activities will stimulate my brain enough to keep me awake.

July 29, 1953: *It still hasn't fully dawned on me that Carl is so far away for three whole months. I was always elated to have Saturday nights off duty, but last Saturday I dreaded it because I knew I would be lonesome for him.*

As it turned out, I wasn't alone on Saturday night after all. A prominent lawyer's wife called and asked me to care for their little boy that evening. When I got there, she had fed him and put him to bed so all I had to do was be there in case he woke up. I read a book, watched TV, and sewed on the dress I was making. When they returned at 12:15 a.m., they paid me $4.15.

A few days later, I went to Mollie's home to spend the day. I helped Mother bake a big batch of cookies and 5 pies. Yummmmy! It doesn't seem possible that it's going to be my last time at home one of these days. Mother and I talked about how different it will be when student days are over and I start living my new, independent life. I can hardly wait, and yet I do hate to leave all my dear families and friends here. But then, I have so much to look forward to. So I'll just take things as they come.

I came to work that night with no sleep all day. It was a busy night, so I wasn't tempted to get sleepy. It will catch up with me eventually. I have enjoyed this stretch of night duty because I'm feeling much more confident. That was my last shift, and I was pleased when Miss G. gave me a good efficiency rating this time!

Chapter 27
Apartment Hunting

The middle of August, Mrs. K. gave Naomi and I permission to move off campus if we could find an apartment. It would free up dormitory space for the new student probies due to come in September. The hospital would pay our rent from August 15-September 12 (our last official day as students). It sounded like a good deal to us.

The next day, Naomi and I looked at apartments and decided to rent a third floor walk-up apartment two blocks from the hospital for $5 a week from Mrs. R., one of the nurses' aides. It was one nice, spacious room with twin beds and several windows that let in lots of air and sunshine. After three long years, we were eager to spread our wings away from this stuffy place, believe me!

Work again on Men's Surgical Ward

August 10, 1953: *Today I started work on Men's Surgical Ward. Our patients have fractured legs/arms with traction, nasal tubes, and Foley catheters.*

Mr. Fango has third degree burns over a third of his body. He requires lots of pain medication before we change his dressings, and sometimes in between. Nothing is as painful as severe burns and the necessary dressing changes.

Ms. Kasig, the supervisor, is nice to work with now that I'm a senior. I remember what a hard time she gave me as a junior. We have a lot of fun there with two very nice Christian orderlies. What a difference from the ones in the E.R. who tell nasty jokes.

August 13, 1953: *We admitted 18-year-old George who had a head-on collision with a truck. He was really in bad shape – unconscious; fractured skull, jaws, collar bone; many cuts and bruises. He still hasn't regained consciousness. Poor fellow. Sure hope he pulls through. Also, we have Kit Carson, aka "Sunset" Carson who had a career as a movie star several years ago. He was also in a bad* *accident. His pelvis and both legs were fractured. It's a wonder he survived.*

August 15, 1953: *In another month, I'll officially be finished as a student nurse and will be a graduate nurse! What will that be like, I wonder?*

August 17, 1953: *We admitted four new patients plus having two fracture reductions, one colonic irrigation, six IVs to monitor, one clysis (replacing fluid to the body subcutaneously), two cut-downs for IV fluids, and four burn dressing changes to keep us busy.*

The doctor wired poor George's jaws shut today. What a miserable time he's going to have the next couple of weeks while his jaws heal. He can barely suck liquids through a straw.

The ambulance brought in a young man who was driving under the influence of alcohol when he drove off the highway and hit a tree, totaling the vehicle. Unfortunately he was totaled also. No surprise there. With a crushed skull, he was very close to death's door. I didn't think he would live as long as he did. At 4:40 a.m., he died a horrible death. I felt so sorry for his distraught wife and two young children. They took it so hard and cried inconsolably for a long time.

Rodney and I went out with the ambulance to help with a three-car accident on the highway. Two of the victims were admitted on our unit, one with a punctured lung and the other with severe lacerations. The driver of one car died there on the gruesome, gory scene.

Five of us seniors are working on Men's Surgical. The patients give each of us a nickname – they call me Minnie the Missile. We have lots of fun joking with them as we give haircuts and shaves, clip toenails and change surgical/burn dressings.

August 28, 1953: *It is so very hot and sultry we can hardly breathe. I'm glad this is the last summer I have to put up with this sticky state. Men's Surgical is still busy with lots of bed baths, back rubs, bedsores and IV's. Now that we have some decent orderlies it's much more pleasant to work there.*

Moving to the apartment

The day we had planned to move to the apartment, Naomi woke up feeling sick to her stomach and ended up in the infirmary with the flu bug. I packed both her stuff and mine by myself. Then later in the day, her parents came in their car to help take me and all our belongings to the apartment. She was still in the infirmary, hoping to be discharged the next day.

Our large third-floor room was very cozy and comfortable, just the right size for two people. Cheerful pink and white curtains decorated the windows. A fan from home really helped on the hot, humid days when there was very little breeze.

I was lonesome without Naomi, though. We'd been rooming together for two years, so I hardly knew how to act all by myself the first night in our new room. However, I felt so free to be on my own that I danced a little jig right there in the middle of the room. It would be strange not having Mrs. G. come around to collect a fine for some infraction or remind me it was time for lights out.

It was hard to leave my dear classmates after being together, sharing trials and tears for three long years. They had to move out of their dorms, too, and start on their own careers. I wished them great success.

August 20, 1953: *Tomorrow, 77 probationers will begin their next three years of nursing school. More power to them. We thought our class was big with 55. This new group will overwhelm us.*

It feels like I'm already independent. I spent the evening in the apartment reading and writing letters. This week I can have three overnights if I want to. That's almost too good to be true. It will be like another vacation. How wonderful!

September 3, 1953: *The hot, sticky weather makes working on the wards like torture. There's no motivation to do anything. We can hardly breathe. You can't imagine how terrible it is unless you really have to endure it. It's supposed to break tomorrow. There have been 104 deaths in 11 days reported over the nation from heat alone.*

As you can see, things are so dull around here that all I have to report is the weather. What keeps me going is the tingly feeling when I think that I am just days away from being a full-fledged graduate nurse. It's hard to wait.

September 7, 1953: *Sue and I were asked to work 7-11 this morning in addition to a night shift tonight. Now get this - we refused! That's what seniors about to be graduates can do – refuse to work overtime. I'm about to go on night duty again with only two more nights to work in my blue uniform. Then I wear my whites when I go to Maternity next week as a graduate. Oh glory!*

September 8, 1953: *This is my last night in nursing school! The tradition around here is that seniors rip off each other's student uniform into shreds as if it were an old rag. I wish you could have seen my ragged, ripped uniform after my co-workers were done with me. It was unwearable. I had to scrounge around for a scrub gown to wear on duty the rest of the shift.*

Tomorrow night we will wear our white uniforms when we go to work. Oh HAPPY NIGHT! Just think, I'll be working for pay then – $1.15 an hour. That will sure feel different.

[Author's note: When I retired in 1995 I was making $18 an hour. What a difference.]

On my last night on Men's Surgical Ward, it was hard to say goodbye knowing I'd never see them again. I really loved it there this time and became very attached to the patients. Two years before, though, I didn't love it. Time and more experience made the difference.

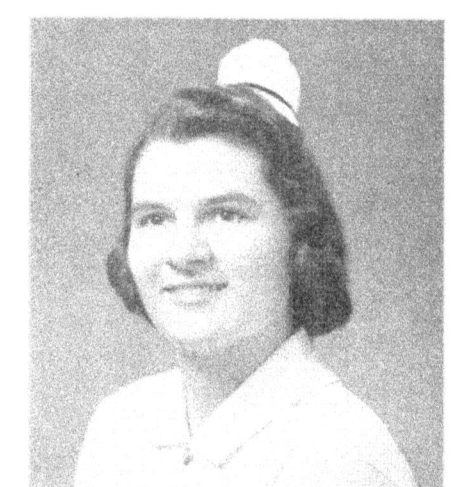

Marilyn at graduation

Chapter 28
Employed in Labor and Delivery; State Boards

September 18, 1953: *I'm still getting used to the idea of freedom. It became reality, though, on Tuesday when I got my first pay check. It was for $38.00 for 4 days of work. Not bad, eh?*

If I wasn't so lazy this week, I would have written in my journal sooner. I have no studies, nothing to force me to structure my time now. I've been really neglectful lately, so I must catch up. This record proves too interesting to discontinue, especially since I'm free at last.

September 29, 1953: *I'm still getting used to the idea of being a regular employee of the hospital working on the Maternity Ward in Preemie Nursery. The babies are so TINY. Rosie and I brought our funniest jokes to tell each other while we fed the babies. How we laughed at our own silliness. I thought I could hear the babies laugh, too.*

This week, Miss R. has assigned me to mentor the junior nursing students on 3rd Floor Maternity so they get experience on a private room floor.

October 6, 1953: *The labor and delivery rooms were all full last night. Seven fathers were so nervous and antsy, pacing up and down in the hallways at one time, waiting for news about their wives and newborn babies.*

A couple of weeks ago, I wrote to Mrs. Hanard, the director of the hospital in my hometown, to inquire about jobs there after November 1. Today I received an answer from her saying she only has one staff nurse vacancy – 3-11. Now isn't that ducky? I'm sick of evening shift. I won't work that shift. I won't…I won't…I won't!

October 20, 1953: *I overslept yesterday and didn't arrive in time for work at 11 p.m. Since our landlady doesn't have a telephone in her house, Miss M., my supervisor, had to call the police to come get me. Mrs. R. was shocked when she answered the knock at the door at 11:30 p.m. There stood a policeman asking for Miss Minter. I was so* *embarrassed. Everyone at work got a big kick out of this incident and teased me mercilessly. After this experience, Mrs. R. had a phone installed. Good idea.*

Just think, only seven more days to work here. On my time off I have been studying diligently for state boards. Three years ago I thought that State Boards were terribly far away. You better believe I'll miss those paychecks for a while until I start a new job.

After visiting and saying goodbyes to my friends in Philadelphia over the weekend, I dashed madly to get the 4:20 p.m. train in order to attend my farewell party at the church before the Sunday evening service. The train pulled away just as I arrived at the station. Drats! I bawled right then and there. I was so heartbroken. I called the pastor at church to let him know I wouldn't make it in time for the party my friends had planned for me at the church. So I waited (not so patiently) for the 5:40 p.m. train. Instead, we had the party after the service. It was hard to say goodbye to all my dear friends there at the church.

Taking State Board Exams

The end of October, I packed up all my stuff. The time had really come to leave this place where I have laughed, loved, and lived for three years. I didn't know if I could sleep, though, thinking about the tough tests coming up. The intense dread of the State Boards left me feeling very jittery. Just the thought of them was a terrible weight on me. Would all my studying pay off? I was counting on it. My future hung on how well I performed on these tests, the last hurdle to jump over before being granted the coveted Registered Nurse (RN) license. By successfully passing those exams, I could legally put those magic initials after my name and be professionally equipped to enter the rough-and-tumble workaday medical world.

October 30-31, 1953: *The State Board of Nursing Exam was given over a two day period in one of the office buildings on the State Capitol campus in Harrisburg. For two days, graduate nurses from across the state sat for eight long hours in the uncomfortable, hard-backed chairs with a 15 minute break in the morning and in the* *evening and an hour for lunch. We slogged through the many pages of multiple choice and essay questions covering all the different subjects we had in classes.*

After the tests were over, there was nothing more to say or do. My poor brain could hardly take any more. It was like a 50- ton weight was lifted off of my shoulders – such a relief! All that was left was the nagging anxiety about whether I had passed or not. But I would have to wait 10 weeks until I was notified of the results.

Carl's parents had arranged to pick me up around 3 p.m. on Saturday, but they misunderstood my directions and were waiting for me at another corner. Finally, after two hours, they drove around looking for me. They found me sitting on the bench where I had told them I'd be waiting. I was a nervous wreck, though, while I waited not knowing what the delay was.

It was 5 p.m. when we started on the long but pleasant trip west to Kansas. With three drivers, it was an easy drive straight through during the 23 hours. Carl was joyfully waiting for us when we pulled up to where he was living in Topeka. It was wonderful to see him again! He showed us around the re-construction project he was working on, and he drove with us to my parents' home where my family hosted all of us royally for two days.

It felt really good to relax and enjoy a whole different lifestyle on the farm with my family. I realized what a terrible tension I had experienced the last few weeks as I studied for the State Board Exams and worked night duty at the same time.

That night, the first snow of the season began with big, fat flakes floating softly down from the sky. For the next two days, everything was draped in a glistening white mantle, so beautiful and peaceful. It seemed to be putting out a welcome mat for me saying, "We're glad you're home again!"

Chapter 29
Start New Job; Receiving License

Interview and Getting Hired

In my interview with Mrs. H., director of nurses at the Abilene Hospital, I remembered that a month before I foolishly vowed up and down I wouldn't work the 3-11 shifts ever again. However, I needed a job and she needed an evening nurse so I agreed to take the 3-11 staff nurse position. She hired me immediately as a graduate nurse (GN). It would take several more weeks to receive my RN license.

Mrs. H. was very pleasant and invited me to have dinner with the other nurses. They gave me royal treatment and accepted me into the staff family. It was a small, rural hospital only nine miles from home, but I felt good about working there. With only around 30 beds, it would be a huge change from the 450-bed LGH facility.

When I returned home from the interview, Mom said I had gotten two calls from someone at the other hospital where I had applied. The nurse there wanted me to work full time 3-11 also. I took this as a definite sign that I was to be at Abilene Hospital. Who knows, had I been home, I might have accepted that job 30 miles away. I began working at the Abilene Hospital a week later.

In starting new jobs, my colleagues and I discovered that in the real world of hospitals and clinics certain procedures were done differently than how we had been so methodically taught by our instructors and supervisors; we would be expected to adapt to our employers' ways of doing things. For some of us freshly minted nurses, that disconnect would prove frustrating. Flexibility became the name of the game.

Getting State Board Exam Results

It was a bittersweet day in January, 1954, when I was notified that I had successfully passed all of the State Board tests except Pediatrics and Psychiatry. I was terribly disappointed, frustrated, and humiliated.

They were scheduled to be given again in April, so I would need to return to Pennsylvania to re-take those two tests.
With that major wrinkle to consider, Carl wrapped up his work in Topeka and we planned our wedding for the end of March. We drove back to Pennsylvania so I could re-take those tests. What a thing to have to do on our wedding trip! It was somewhat comforting to discover that I wasn't alone. Seventeen of my classmates also were there to re-take them. I didn't feel quite so embarrassed, after all.

In June, I was notified that I had successfully passed the tests. Now that was something to crow about. A couple of weeks later, I received an oblong piece of stiff, embossed paper – my cherished Pennsylvania nursing license for which I had worked three long, arduous years. It was thrilling to know that now I was a full-fledged licensed registered nurse. My heart overflowed with gratitude. Tears of relief and joy ran down my cheeks.

A Poem

Ode to an Embossed Piece of Paper: Letting Go of My Nursing License

A mere sixty five years ago
This naïve nineteen year old began
Her long, arduous journey.
She didn't know how hard it would be
To follow her dream to become a nurse.

As the path grew steeper
Trials and tears soon followed;
Faith often fought with fatigue.
Could she endure to the end?

She gained confidence
In her skills and knowledge;
Some patients got well, some didn't.
In spite of it all she never gave up her dream.

That embossed piece of paper
Would tell the whole world
She had indeed climbed the rugged mountain,
Reached the peak and received her nursing license!
What a thrill to put those coveted Initials
After her name in a patient's progress chart!
"RN" for registered nurse.
That person is me.

After sixty five years of toil and moil
The time has come to say goodbye
To that embossed piece of paper
That I worked so hard for.
I relinquished my nursing license this year,
Let it lapse and let it go – forever.
It was just a piece of embossed paper
But oh it held so many memories!

Now at eighty five years old
My identity as a registered nurse is history.
No more paychecks for me.
I will always be a nurse in spirit.
Care for hurting, dying people will never leave me.
I weep for my loss,
But at the same time,
I remember with pride,
It's been an amazing ride!

Marilyn Minter Wolgemuth, December 2015

Epilogue

In March, 1954, Carl and I were married in the little country church near my home where I had grown up. We immediately took up another voluntary service assignment ministering to agricultural migrants in Fresno County, California.

In the 61 years since then, I have been blessed with a wide variety of experiences in my nursing career: hospital staff nurse, public health nurse, maternity, labor and delivery, school nurse, doctor's clinic nurse manager, and psychiatric nurse/counselor in a mental health hospital.

For several years, my husband and I lived and worked with an indigenous Aztec group under the Wycliffe Bible Translators Mission. I was the only professional medical person within a 50 mile radius in a remote, mountainous, tropical area of southern Mexico. There were no modern medical services there, so I was able to learn and analyze the unwritten Nahuatl language, provide basic medical care, and provide health teaching in addition to homeschooling our daughter through seventh grade.

In 1970-71, we took a year's furlough from our mission work and I returned to Messiah College for my Bachelor of Science in Nursing degree that was just beginning to be offered.

In 1974, we left the tropics and settled near the Wycliffe headquarters in Dallas, Texas. I was asked to take charge of setting up a health clinic on the campus to provide a wide range of services for returning and outgoing missionaries. I soon realized that those who came for help at the clinic had emotional as well as physical needs. In order to minister there more effectively, I knew I needed more training in counseling. So at age 50, I graduated magna cum laude with a Bachelor of Science degree in psychology and counseling from Dallas Baptist University. It was a stimulating experience to be in classes with 18-25 year olds!

From 1981until my retirement in 1995, I worked in the mental health field, including five years in a hospital addictions unit. After I retired, I kept my nursing license active and did volunteer nursing for the next twenty years. A nurse friend and I started a healthcare ministry in our church where I served as one of the parish nurses for several years.

My RN license needed to be renewed every two years, so in 2015, at age 85, I vacillated back and forth about whether or not to renew it. After much thought, I decided it was time to give it up – the hard-earned treasure that has been a symbol of my professional identity for sixty five years. It proved less difficult than I thought it would be. I'm still a nurse at heart; it's just that I am not licensed to work as a professional nurse anymore. It is with pleasure and satisfaction that I can reflect on a 65-year career I could only dream about when I was 11 years old. What a ride it has been!

Appendix 1: Nursing Education Today

This narrative provides a window into a bygone era so readers will understand how nursing education has changed in the last six and a half decades. Three-year, hospital-based diploma programs are being phased out and are expanding to the multi-level nursing education system we have today. Students wanting to enter the nursing profession can choose to begin at the LPN or ADN/RN level and move up the professional ladder:

- a 12- to 18-month course for Licensed Practical or Vocational Nurses (LPN/LVN)
- a two-year program that grants ADN/RN (Associate Degree /Registered Nurse)
- Four-year colleges now offer the Bachelor of Science in Nursing (BSN) or an accelerated RN-BSN program
- a Master of Science in Nursing (MSN)
- a Doctor of Nursing Practice (DNP).

There are other specialty nursing degrees such as Advanced Practice Registered Nurse (APRN) in addition to the above major programs. An APRN is a nurse who has a master's or post-master's certificate in a particular specialty. In some states, APRNs can generally practice medicine without the supervision of a physician. Nurse practitioners, Nurse anesthetists, Nurse midwives, and clinical nurse specialists are all considered APRNs.

Recently I shared some of my student experiences with a young friend who graduated from the two-year ADN/RN program four years ago. She expressed feeling a bit of envy because I had received so many more extensive clinical experiences than she did before she graduated. She said that in general, today's newly graduated nurses are able to sharpen their clinical expertise only during and after their first job orientation.

As I spoke with this young nurse, I became very grateful for the education and practical experiences that transformed my dream of becoming a nurse into a vocation that served me well during the next six and a half decades.

Appendix 2: Men Join the Nursing Profession

Traditionally, only women were admitted to the rigorous academic nursing programs, however CBS News carried this news item on February 26, 2013:

"Men, in fact, had been largely kept out of nursing in past decades because nursing schools often refused to admit men. The Supreme Court ruled that practice was unconstitutional in 1981 after a case involving a state nursing school."

"In the 1970s 2.7 percent of registered nurses were men. A new study from the United States Census Bureau tracked data through 2011 and reported the number of male nurses has more than tripled. The study found that men now make up 9.6 percent of all employed registered nurses (RNs) in the United States totaling about 330,000 men in total. The report also noted the proportion of licensed male practical and vocational nurses (LPNs and LVNs) has more than doubled since 1970 from 3.9 percent to 8.1 percent."

"Men were found to be more likely to become nurse anesthetists which is the highest paid nursing occupation, and were found least likely to become LPNs or LVNs (licensed practical or licensed vocational nurses), the lowest paid type of nursing."

Appendix 3: About Lancaster General Hospital

Important historical information about LGH is available from a pictorial account written by Harold J. Eager in 1993 for the 100th anniversary – 100 years of caring: Lancaster General Hospital. Forward thinking citizens of Lancaster founded the hospital with the first patient in a building on Queen Street in 1893. Three nursing students were accepted that year. The School of Nursing formally began 10 years later, in 1903. In 1910, 30 student nurses were enrolled. The hospital has expanded steadily and extensively from that small beginning to what it is today.

In 1950, the hospital census was 285 patients. A new addition opened in 1952 that added 156 additional beds. With several additions since then, including two other locations, it has grown to a total of 690 beds.

The LGH School of Nursing is now called Pennsylvania College of Health Sciences. The 2015-2016 winter issue of the *InPractice*, the college magazine reports, that 1400 students are enrolled in more than 24 health science programs. Allied medical services such as X-Ray technician, Emergency medical technician, and laboratory technician are among the programs offered today.

This recent news item on April 21, 2015, further updates the institution:

Lancaster General Health (LG Health) and the University of Pennsylvania Health System (Penn Medicine) jointly approved an agreement today to have LG Health become a member of Penn Medicine. (www.lancastergeneralhealth.org/LGH/about and http://www.lancastergeneralhealth.org/LGH/News-Home/News-Room/News-Releases/2015/Lancaster-General-Health-decides-to-join-Universit.aspx).

I am very pleased to be a graduate of this prestigious institution.

Other books by Carl and Marilyn Minter Wolgemuth

- *The "Ideal" Couple: The Shadow Side of a Marriage.*
  Cascadia Publishing, 2010.

- *God's Talk: Bringing the Gospel to the Isthmus Aztecs of Mexico in Their Heart Language.*
  Self-published, 2012.

- *Barefoot Girl: The Childhood Memoirs of a Kansas Sunflower.*
  Self-published, 2015.

All are available on Amazon.com or at bookstores.

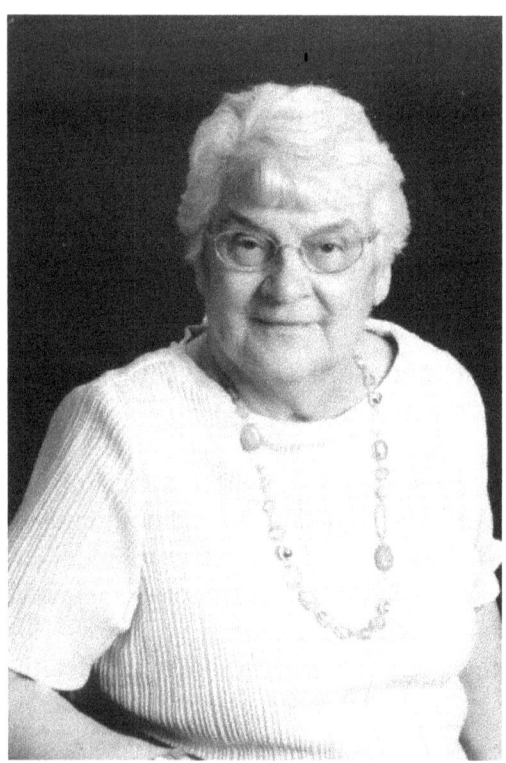

Marilyn Joyce Minter Wolgemuth

www.ingramcontent.com/pod-product-compliance
Lightning Source LLC
Chambersburg PA
CBHW050459110426
42742CB00018B/3314